W9-CNF-315

RUNNING/TRACK & FIELD

"My athletes already follow the principles outlined in *The Performance Zone* to great success."
JOE VIGIL, PH.D., CO-HEAD COACH, TEAM USA CALIFORNIA

"I am hoping my competition doesn't read *The Performance Zone*."
LORNAH KIPLAGAT, WORLD-RECORD HOLDER

"From now on, *The Performance Zone* will be required reading for all of the athletes I coach."
FRANK GAGLIANO, HEAD COACH, NIKE FARM TEAM

"*The Performance Zone* covers not only the what and why, but also the all-important 'how to.' It's cutting edge."
ROY BENSON, M.P.E., PRIVATE RUNNING COACH

"This is the best nutrition book for runners I have ever read."
JEFF GALLOWAY, AUTHOR OF *GALLOWAY'S BOOK ON RUNNING*

TRIATHLON

"Whether you're an aspiring soccer player or dreaming of racing in the Tour de France, this book is an absolute must for your health library."
DAVE SCOTT, SIX-TIME WINNER, HAWAII IRONMAN

"*The Performance Zone* takes all of the guesswork out of sports nutrition."
SIRI LINDLEY, #1 WORLD RANKED TRIATHLETE, 2001–2003

"*The Performance Zone* is an incredible coaching tool."
TROY JACOBSON, FOUNDER AND PRESIDENT, THE TRIATHLON ACADEMY

CYCLING/MOUNTAIN BIKING

"This is the most valuable and practical book on how nutrition can improve sports performance."
ANDY PRUITT, ED.D., FOUNDER, BOULDER CENTER FOR SPORTS MEDICINE

"*The Performance Zone* is that rare book valuable both to the professional athlete and the beginner."
RYDER HESJEDAL, 2002 NORBA SERIES CHAMPION

"*The Performance Zone* is a fantastic and much needed resource that every athlete, regardless of sport or ability level, should take full advantage of. I wouldn't break another sweat without first reading this book!"
ALISON DUNLAP, 2001 MOUNTAIN BIKE WORLD CHAMPION

SOCCER

"Any athlete, regardless of age, who implements *The Performance Zone* action plan will experience a quantum leap in performance."
JOSH WOLFF, U.S. NATIONAL TEAM MEMBER

"Drs. Ivy and Portman's book will give every player, parent, and coach the necessary information to go into competition with an edge."

DON KIRKENDALL, PH.D.,
MEMBER OF THE U.S. SOCCER
SPORTS MEDICINE COMMITTEE

HOCKEY

"Drs. Portman and Ivy are not only at the cutting edge of sports nutrition— they define the cutting edge."

PAUL GOLDBERG, R.D., C.S.C.S.,
STRENGTH AND CONDITIONING COACH,
COLORADO AVALANCHE

"I have waited a long time for a book like *The Performance Zone*. It fulfills an important need for athletes, coaches, and parents."

KIRK OLSON, DIRECTOR OF STRENGTH
AND CONDITIONING, MINNESOTA WILD

"This book provides a practical guide to sports nutrition that can be utilized by hockey players at all levels."

JIM RAMSAY, ATHLETIC TRAINER,
NEW YORK RANGERS

"*The Performance Zone* is the crucial nutritional blueprint to help athletes perform at their best mentally and physically."

MIKE RICHTER, FORMER NHL ALL STAR
AND USA OLYMPIC TEAM GOALIE

BASKETBALL

"*The Performance Zone* will help my players get that edge everyone is searching for. It will give us the nutritional guidelines to be able to train harder in our quest for the NBA title."

RICH DALATRI, C.S.C.S., STRENGTH
AND CONDITIONING COACH,
NEW JERSEY NETS

FOOTBALL

"*The Performance Zone* will become the nutrition bible for football players and coaches."

JON TORINE, STRENGTH AND
CONDITIONING COACH,
INDIANAPOLIS COLTS

LACROSSE

"Practicing the sports nutrition methods described in *The Performance Zone* has made me a better athlete, plain and simple."

A. J. HAUGEN, THREE-TIME
MLL ALL-STAR

SWIMMING

"*The Performance Zone* will make an immediate difference in helping you reach your potential."

JOSH DAVIS, FIVE-TIME OLYMPIC
MEDAL WINNER

THE PERFORMANCE ZONE

Your Nutrition Action Plan for Greater Endurance & Sports Performance

John Ivy, Ph.D. & Robert Portman, Ph.D.

Foreword by Dave Scott, Six-Time Winner Hawaii Ironman

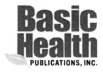

Basic Health PUBLICATIONS, INC.

The information contained in this book is based upon the research and personal and professional experiences of the authors. It is not intended as a substitute for consulting with your physician or other healthcare provider. Any attempt to diagnose and treat an illness should be done under the direction of a healthcare professional.

The publisher does not advocate the use of any particular healthcare protocol but believes the information in this book should be available to the public. The publisher and authors are not responsible for any adverse effects or consequences resulting from the use of the suggestions, preparations, or procedures discussed in this book. Should the reader have any questions concerning the appropriateness of any procedures or preparation mentioned, the authors and the publisher strongly suggest consulting a professional healthcare advisor.

Basic Health Publications, Inc.
28812 Top of the World Drive
Laguna Beach, CA 92651
Phone: 949-715-7327

Library of Congress Cataloging-in-Publication Data

Ivy, John.
   The performance zone : your nutrition action plan for greater endurance and sports performance / John Ivy and Robert Portman ; foreword by Dave Scott.
      p. cm. — (Teen health series)
   Includes bibliographical references and index.
   ISBN 1-59120-148-9
  1. Athletes—Nutrition. I. Portman, Robert. II. Title. III. Series.

   TX361.A8I984   2004
   613.2'024'796—dc22

                                                          2004005397

Copyright © 2004 John Ivy, Ph.D., and Robert Portman, Ph.D.

All rights reserved. No part of this publication may be reproduced, stored in a retrieval system, or transmitted, in any form or by any means, electronic, mechanical, photocopying, recording, or otherwise, without the prior written consent of the copyright owner.

Editor: Carol Rosenberg
Typesetter/Book design: Gary A. Rosenberg
Cover design: Mike Stromberg

Images on pages 12, 20, 31, 32, 34, 40, 43, 49, 50, 51, 76, 77, 78, 79, 80, 82, 83, 85, 88, 89, 91, 92, 93, 94, 95, 98, 99 copyright © 1997 PhotoDisc, Inc.

Printed in the United States of America

10   9   8   7   6   5   4   3   2

Contents

Acknowledgments

Our goal was to write a useful, easy-to-read book based on the latest science that all athletes, regardless of sport, will find valuable. If we achieve that goal, our gratitude goes out to the many experts we consulted—including Dave Scott, Kim Brown, Rich Dalatri, Josh Davis, Alison Dunlap, Jeff Galloway, Paul Goldberg, A. J. Haugen, Dr. Don Kirkendall, Siri Lindley, Dr. Nanna Meyers, Andrew Pruitt, Dr. John Seifert, Dr. Jeff Stout, Jon Torine, and Joe Vigil—for their contributions and invaluable suggestions. Special thanks to Matt Fitzgerald for his comments and editorial expertise.

Thanks to the people at Basic Health Publications, particularly Carol and Gary Rosenberg—the best possible book-production team any writer could want—for making sure this book was published on time despite another impossible schedule.

And thanks to the late Dr. Ed Burke, whose enthusiasm, knowledge, and dedication to sport continues to inspire us.

Most of all, we wish to acknowledge the hundreds of researchers whose studies form the backbone of this book and the many athletes who encouraged us to write a simple, practical tool that athletes, coaches, and parents of athletes in all sports can use.

Finally, a special thank you to our wives, Susan and Jennifer, for serving as sounding boards, for their patience, and most of all, for their encouragement.

Foreword

was watching a triathlete struggling to complete last year's Ironman race and asked her what she ate during the bike and run segments. "Chocolate, just chocolate bars!" she replied. After nearly thirty years competing as a triathlete and now as a coach, my simple response to this triathlete was, "There are better choices!"

Endurance athletes have always tried to find the "magic food" or the "secret" training and racing beverage that would extend or possibly accelerate their performance. Despite the wealth of information regarding carbohydrate fluid replacement drinks, there has always been a cloud of confusion deciphering the fueling for endurance activities. Unraveling this nutritional puzzle has been extremely confounding. The myths and misconceptions of fueling for endurance events present a host of questions: What foods/fluids are the best choices for exercise? How can my recovery be enhanced if I take in calories after exercise? Will I be able to train longer and harder with proper fueling?

The complexity of these questions seemingly stymies the endurance athlete with too many nutritional unknowns.

Closing the loop from world-class competitors to the recreational athlete, the authors of *The Performance Zone*, Drs. Portman and Ivy, have masterfully woven the complexities of fueling for endurance. Extracting from research and practical application, this book streamlines the application of fueling your system before, during, and after exercise.

The notion of just taking in a few carbohydrates for exercise is no longer valid. *The Performance Zone* has taken the guesswork out of muscle fueling. Drs. Portman and Ivy have extrapolated and condensed their information so the reader can selectively extract and apply their personal nutritional concerns.

Why is this book different from any other nutritional book or manual? Following are just a few of the "secrets" within the chapters. First, this is the only book that properly correlates the type of fuel before, during, and after exercise. For example, protein must be combined with carbohydrate to maximize the response of the hormone insulin. Carbo-

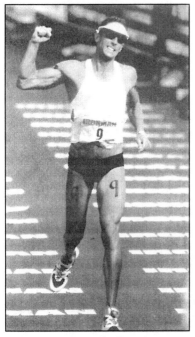

Dave Scott

hydrate alone is not nearly as effective as the combination of the two. The fueling mix must be consumed at all three phases. Second, the immune system is greatly enhanced by the consumption of the proper balance of nutrients, again, before, during, and after exercise. The underlying theme is that when the nutrients are timed properly, the body will adapt and respond more effectively. Third, endurance athletes are always trying to repair, rebuild, and recover from day to day. *The Performance Zone* has an exact formula for nutritional rebuilding and recovering that can be implemented for your specific weight, intensity, and duration of exercise. This is the only book that precisely describes this methodology.

In *The Performance Zone,* through impeccable research and simple practical guidelines, you will be able to construct the ideal nutrition plan for yourself. This book is truly the most comprehensive compilation of athletic fueling. Whether you're an aspiring soccer player or dreaming of racing in the Tour de France, this book is an absolute must for your health library. Read it and reap the benefits.

—Dave Scott, Six-Time Ironman Champion

Introduction

We frequently lecture to athletes, coaches, and parents on the importance of nutrition in improving sports performance. After our lectures, we are always bombarded with questions from our audience. Which nutrients are best to eat before, during, and after exercise? How often should one drink during exercise? How much? Is water sufficient?

From the large number and types of questions we get, it's apparent that there is an "information disconnect" between the science of sports nutrition and the fields, arenas, roads, pools, and gyms where athletes perform. The causes of this disconnect are multiple. Some people are getting too little information, and some are getting too much. Most are getting dated and conflicting information often colored by marketing hype.

For adult athletes who religiously read their monthly sports-specific magazines, the disconnect is caused by an information overload. In a desire to give their subscribers new reasons to read each month, magazines dispense information on nutrition that promises too much, is touted as "the next big breakthrough," and often contradicts the previous month's article. Serious athletes who are looking for solid information must try to separate fact from fiction. Since most athletes have no formal background in nutrition or exercise physiology, this presents quite a challenge.

For the coach (especially of young athletes), the problem is different. Coaches have so many responsibilities—scheduling, training, developing travel schedules, and so forth—that proper nutrition is almost totally neglected or taken for granted. This is unfortunate, since coaches are the major source of information on nutrition for young athletes. Coaches need practical information that their athletes can understand, and it's hard to find.

For the parent of young athletes, the problem is usually a lack of information. General nutrition articles that appear in the popular media may not be relevant to the special needs of young athletes. And, in fact, some of the popular nutrition fads, such as the current low-carbohydrate diets, may actually be detrimental to a child's athletic performance.

Not all athletes are faced with this problem. Most professional teams and athletes either have a personal nutritionist or have access to a team nutritionist who works with the strength coach to develop individualized nutrition programs. Unfortunately, a personal nutritionist is a luxury few athletes can afford.

The Performance Zone—Your Own Sports Nutritionist

This book provides a simple, effective nutrition action plan for every athlete, and for the coaches and parents who guide them. This action plan is specific to the period we refer to as the "Performance Zone," beginning about a half hour before training and competition, extending through the practice or competition, and ending shortly after the practice or competition. In other words, this is not a book of general dietary guidelines for athletes. There are already many books that handle this topic adequately. Performance Zone nutrition is an issue unto itself, and one that requires special attention—from all athletes.

The action plan described in this book is built on science—not just the results of a single study, but the consensus of hundreds of studies from leading sports science laboratories around the world. We have converted this information into a few basic strategies that athletes can use to raise their level of athletic performance.

We also recognize that these universal nutritional guidelines must be adapted and customized to individual sports in order to accommodate their unique requirements. To this end, we have called on the expertise of Olympic athletes, leading exercise physiologists, coaches, and nutritionists, who have provided sport-specific nutrition tips for all of the major sports.

Our Guarantee

Although we are scientists, we would like to make every reader a guarantee. We realize this may sound very commercial. Scientists usually don't make guarantees. But in this case, the scientific facts themselves allow us to guarantee that if you incorporate the Performance Zone action plan into your own training program, your team's training program, or your child's training program, you will see a significant improvement in athletic performance.

Only a small fraction of athletes at any level are currently practicing the best and most cutting-edge sport nutrition methods described in this book, or anything remotely like them. This is another reason we feel confident making the promise that significant performance enhancement will come with adopting these methods.

We are not suggesting that the Performance Zone action plan will make you or the athletes you train into Olympic gold medalists. There is much more that goes into athletic performance than nutrition. Training, commitment, genetics, talent, and will are essential factors to reach elite status in any sport. However, whatever your level of athletic performance, the nutrition action plan described in this book can help you reach your full potential.

1.
The Performance Zone

A rticles on sports nutrition in the mainstream media usually contain a quote from a nutritionist that goes something like this: "For optimal performance, athletes only need a healthy, natural-food, high-carbohydrate diet and plenty of fluid during exercise." We agree that a healthy diet is essential for athletes (as it is for everyone else). However, ignoring the increased nutrient requirements of athletes borders on irresponsible. Hundreds of studies have documented the fact that athletes require additional nutrients during exercise to optimize their performance.

But the primary reason we take such strong issue with the dismissal of specialized exercise nutrition is that it ignores the relationship between fueling muscles during exercise and the development of muscle fatigue and the relationship between muscle fatigue and injuries.

Over the past ten years, research reinforced by the experience of athletes and coaches has demonstrated that tired athletes are injured more frequently because their reaction times and mental perceptions are slowed. In almost every team sport, the incidence of injuries increases in the latter stages of competition when athletes are tired. Sports training places special demands on the muscles and other systems of the body. A healthy diet is certainly the appropriate foundation for an athlete's overall nutrition regimen, but it is only a foundation. To maximize energy and minimize the risk of injury during exercise, and to recover quickly and adapt fully after exercise, athletes must be proactive in feeding their muscles during and after exercise.

This concept is not new. In the 1950s and 1960s (and, incredibly, sometimes even today), coaches practiced the theory that withholding water made athletes "tougher." More often, it sent them to the hospital, or even to the morgue. In response, concerned exercise physiologists and nutritionists implemented awareness programs for coaches around the country in which they taught the importance of consuming water during exercise to prevent heat illness and improve athletic performance.

In the 1970s, researchers at the Human Performance Laboratory at Ball State University began publishing studies on the effect of carbohydrate supplementation during exercise on athletic performance. This research started the sports drink revolution. Many studies were published documenting the fact that carbohydrate, when combined with fluid, reduces muscle fatigue and improves athletic performance in almost every sport. "Carbo-loading" became part of the popular nomenclature as athletes sought new ways to increase their muscle energy stores to improve performance. Pasta replaced steak as the pre-event meal of choice. For the endurance athlete and the team sports athlete alike, carbohydrate and fluid must be the two cornerstones of exercise nutrition.

In the past decade, there has been another quiet revolution taking place in sports science laboratories around the world. It is a revolution that will change sports nutrition practices forever. The results from this research are testing some of our long-held beliefs about what constitutes the ideal nutrients during exercise. *The Performance Zone* will show you how to incorporate this science into your own program to improve your athletic performance. It will also challenge many of the myths and misconceptions you've probably been exposed to. Let's take a look at the science backing this revolution in light of three misconceptions regarding exercise nutrition.

MISCONCEPTION #1
For exercise lasting fewer than forty-five minutes, water is fine.

This is true for low-intensity exercise. However, nutrient requirements during exercise are not only a function of exercise *duration* but also of exercise *intensity*. Although our bodies have sufficient energy to exercise at low to moderate intensities for up to three hours, at high intensities, this energy reservoir may last only thirty minutes. Therefore, high-intensity exercise, even if it lasts only forty-five minutes, requires more than just water.

MISCONCEPTION #2
I have eighteen to twenty hours after my workout to restore my muscles.

Research now shows that in actual time you have only about forty-five minutes after a hard workout or practice to optimally replenish your stores of muscle glycogen (the stored form of carbohydrate) and halt the cellular damage that occurs as a natural consequence of exercise. Consumption of the right nutrients within forty-five minutes after you exercise can dramatically improve how your muscles recover and, most important, how they perform the next time you work out.

MISCONCEPTION #3
Carbohydrate is the nutrient for aerobic athletes; protein is the nutrient for strength athletes and bodybuilders.

This misconception is driven by the media as well as by the manufacturers of carbohydrate sports drinks and protein supplements. There is no doubt that aerobic athletes require more carbohydrate than strength athletes. However, we are now discovering that the addition of protein to a carbohydrate supplement offers significant benefits to aerobic athletes. A carbohydrate/protein supplement can extend endurance more than a carbohydrate-only supplement can. And the addition of protein can have a dramatic impact on the degree of muscle damage and the speed with which the muscles of aerobic athletes recover following a hard workout. Conversely, the addition of carbohydrate to a protein supplement is beneficial to the strength athlete because it stimulates protein synthesis and muscle development to a far greater extent than protein alone.

THE PERFORMANCE ZONE

Most athletes believe that their fitness improves during exercise. But they are only partly correct. Yes, during training, the muscles are primed for adaptations that result in improved strength, power, and endurance. But the actual adaptations occur during recovery, and the extent of these adaptations is highly influenced by both exercise and postexercise nutrition.

In a world of $150 basketball shoes and $500 downloadable heart-rate monitors, athletes tend to focus on how the latest technology in equipment or training might improve performance. Nutrition as a training tool is decidedly low-tech, and for this reason, it doesn't get the attention it deserves. There is nothing special about eating. We do it all the time, whether or not we're athletes. And while most athletes recognize the importance of nutrition on an intellectual level, this awareness is not implemented into their training regimen on a regular basis. All too often, for example, athletes are very particular about their pre-competition meals, but they don't put a moment's thought or planning into recovery nutrition after everyday training.

This book is about using nutrition within the Performance Zone, the period beginning thirty minutes before exercise, continuing throughout exercise, and ending fifteen minutes after exercise. Science clearly shows that the right combination of fluid and nutrients consumed within the Performance Zone will help you improve your athletic performance far more than the latest high-tech equipment or training device. The following are a few basic principles of the Performance Zone that you should understand before we get into the details.

Timing Is Everything

The ability of the muscle machinery to regenerate itself decreases very rapidly after a workout, so that nutrients consumed more than forty-five minutes after exercise will have far less impact in helping the muscles regenerate than nutrients consumed earlier. This may seem contrary to what you would expect. Why should it make any difference *when* you eat as long as you consume the right nutrients before your next game or workout? The answer is that the same nutrients can have very different effects in the body depending on the status of the muscles and blood at the time the nutrients are consumed. And it so happens that immediately after exercise, specifically within fifteen minutes, the status of the muscles and blood is such that, if the right nutrients are consumed, the biochemical regulators of muscle recovery are stimulated more strongly than at any other time. We'll take a closer look at this phenomenon in Chapter 4.

More Is Not Necessarily Better

The second important principle is "nutrient optimization." This principle stresses the importance of consuming just the right balance and combinations of specific nutrients before, during, and after exercise to meet the body's most significant needs at these times. Too many athletes are inclined to follow a contrary "more is better" principle. For example, we know that carbohydrate plays an essential role in delaying fatigue during aerobic exercise. So, one might ask, why not take in even more carbohydrate during exercise for even more energy? This won't work, as you will see in Chapter 3, because of limitations on the body's ability to absorb carbohydrate and also limitations on the muscles' ability to convert carbohydrate into the necessary energy to drive muscle contraction.

It Takes More Than Carbs and Fluid

Within the Performance Zone, the muscles marshal multiple physiological and biochemical systems to produce the necessary energy during exercise and to rebuild and refuel following exercise. Table 1.1 on page 10 details the many factors that nutrient and fluid intervention must address. As you will discover, you need more than carbohydrate and water if you are going to use nutrition to its fullest. For example, the addition of protein and specific vitamins to carbohydrate and water will not only enable you to improve endurance by sparing muscle glycogen stores, but will also enable you to reduce muscle damage and improve muscular endurance in your next exercise session.

The 30W15 Rule

The "30W15 rule" is not a new product that will prevent hinges from squeaking. Rather, it is the heart of the Performance Zone action plan for every athlete, regardless of whether you are an Olympian, a weekend warrior, or a twelve-year-old soccer player. Very simply, the 30W15 rule is an easy way to reinforce the Performance Zone. It stands for starting nutrient intervention 30 minutes before exercise and continuing through your Workout and consuming your recovery nutrition within 15 minutes after your workout. Complying with the 30W15 rule means not only changing your exercise nutrition behavior, but also redefining when your workout begins and when your workout ends.

SUMMARY

The Performance Zone is the time period surrounding your exercise in which nutrient intervention can significantly improve athletic performance. Cutting-edge research from leading exercise physiology

1.1. PERFORMANCE ZONE NUTRITION

Interval	Nutrient Objectives
30 Minutes Before Exercise	• Fully hydrate
	• Raise blood glucose levels
During Exercise	• Replace fluid and electrolytes
	• Preserve muscle glycogen
	• Maintain blood glucose levels
	• Minimize cortisol increases
	• Set the stage for a faster recovery
Within 15 Minutes After Exercise	• Shift the metabolic machinery into an anabolic (muscle-building) state from a catabolic (muscle-depleting) state
	• Replenish muscle glycogen stores
	• Initiate tissue repair and set the stage for muscle growth
	• Reduce muscle damage and support the immune system
	• Start the replenishment of fluid and electrolytes

laboratories now shows that consuming the right combination of nutrients before, during, and immediately after exercise can improve endurance, reduce muscle damage, help maintain immune function, and stimulate a much faster recovery.

To appreciate how the Performance Zone can help you become a better athlete, it is important that you understand how muscles use nutrients for energy during exercise, and the consequences of energy production. In the next chapter, we discuss the different energy systems available to the muscles to generate energy and the limitations of each.

2.
Working
Muscles

D uring exercise, the muscles' first priority is to generate the large amounts of energy necessary to drive muscle contractions. In order to produce energy rapidly and efficiently, the muscles must produce and deliver the correct amount of fuel and maintain the right metabolic environment. This requires the synchronization of multiple physiological and biochemical pathways.

Muscles are often compared to the engine of a car. The analogy is quite apt. In order to operate, a car engine requires an uninterrupted supply of fuel delivered to the pistons in a precise way so that it can be converted to energy to drive the wheels. Because internal combustion generates considerable quantities of heat, the engine must be continuously cooled; otherwise, the engine will lock up and stop.

Although the metabolic machinery of your muscles is far more sophisticated than an internal combustion engine, it operates under similar constraints. During exercise, there must be a continuous supply of fuel, the fuel must be converted into a form the muscles can use, and it must be transferred quickly to the pistons of the muscles (muscle fibers) to initiate contraction. The muscle machinery must also be constantly cooled if it is to operate at peak efficiency.

If you view these processes in the context of energy generation, you will easily understand why the right kind of nutrient intervention during exercise can dramatically improve athletic performance.

ENERGY PRODUCTION

Adenosine triphosphate (ATP) is the only source of energy that can drive muscle contraction. ATP is a high-energy phosphate compound.

When ATP is broken down to adenosine diphosphate (ADP) and inorganic phosphate (Pi), energy is released. Interestingly, muscles only store enough ATP for a few seconds of maximal contraction. As a result, ATP must be continuously replenished if muscle contraction is to be sustained. The rate at which ATP must be replenished is directly related to exercise intensity. The greater the exercise intensity, the greater the ATP requirement.

ATP can be produced by three different energy systems, two of which are anaerobic (without oxygen) and one of which is aerobic (with oxygen), as shown in Figure 2.1. The availability of multiple energy systems gives the muscles increased physiological capabilities. For exam-

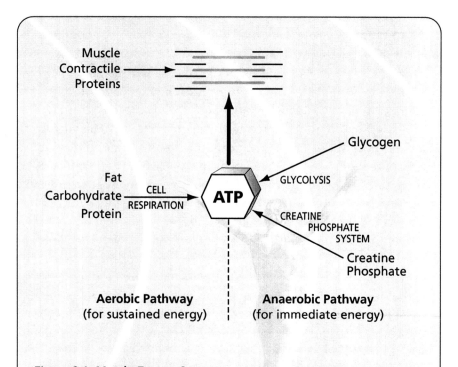

Figure 2.1. Muscle Energy Systems
Because ATP in the muscles is very limited, it must be continuously supplied through both anaerobic and aerobic pathways. The anaerobic pathways provide immediate ATP but in limited amounts and are critical for high-intensity, short-duration exercise. The aerobic pathway provides energy for low- to moderate-intensity exercise, usually of longer duration, by using carbohydrate, fat, and even protein as fuel.

ple, when a soccer player is jogging up and down the field, the energy requirement is low and therefore the primary source of ATP production comes from the aerobic energy system, which is highly efficient. When the soccer player breaks into a sprint to retrieve a loose ball, the ATP required increases quickly, thereby requiring activation of the anaerobic energy systems, which are less efficient but faster.

Anaerobic Energy Production

During high-intensity exercise, your muscles replenish energy through two anaerobic energy systems. The first is the creatine phosphate system. Similar to ATP, creatine phosphate (CP) is a high-energy phosphate compound that supplies energy for the regeneration of ATP. However, as with ATP, the muscle stores of CP are extremely limited. There is only enough CP stored in muscle to support a maximal effort for eight to twelve seconds.

The second anaerobic energy system is glycolysis. Glycolysis generates ATP by the breakdown of carbohydrate stored in the muscles as glycogen and blood glucose. Glycolysis cannot produce ATP as fast as the breakdown of CP, but it is still considerably faster than aerobic energy production. Unfortunately, glycolysis is a relatively inefficient means of producing ATP and one of its byproducts is lactic acid. When lactic acid is produced in high concentrations, it can cause muscle fatigue and adversely affect performance.

Aerobic Energy Production

Aerobic metabolism, or cellular respiration, involves the use of oxygen for ATP production. This process is considerably slower than the anaerobic processes for ATP production but is much more efficient. Cellular respiration as a mechanism of generating ATP is primarily used for exercise intensities that can be sustained for long periods of time such as running a marathon. For most endurance athletes and those who play team sports, aerobic metabolism is the primary source of ATP replenishment.

Aerobic metabolism takes place in small energy-producing factories within the muscle cells called "mitochondria." Mitochondria use oxygen delivered by the circulatory system along with fuels either stored in the muscles or stored elsewhere in the body to generate ATP. The more mitochondria in a muscle, the more efficient the muscle will be in using oxygen to generate ATP.

The limitation of the aerobic energy system is the rate at which oxygen can be delivered to the exercising muscles by the circulatory system. The maximum rate at which oxygen is delivered to the muscles and used for energy is termed "VO_2max."

Exercise intensity is generally defined relative to one's VO_2max. For example, jogging may require an energy expenditure of 50 percent VO_2max, which means that the aerobic energy system needs to function at 50 percent of capacity to generate a sufficient amount of ATP to sustain exercise. As one moves from jogging to running and from running to sprinting, the exercise intensity may increase to 80 percent VO_2max and 130 percent VO_2max, respectively. The ability to run at speeds greater than 100 percent VO_2max is due to our ability to supplement our ATP needs through the anaerobic energy systems. Although anaerobic energy is required for high-intensity exercise and aerobic energy for low- to moderate-intensity exercise, each supports the replenishment of ATP regardless of the exercise intensity. It is only the degree to which each is used that changes as exercise intensity changes.

Unlike the anaerobic energy pathways, which must use either CP or muscle glycogen as fuel to generate ATP, the aerobic energy system can use several different types of fuel. These include carbohydrates in the form of blood glucose and muscle glycogen, fats stored in adipose (fat) and muscle tissue, and amino acids (the building blocks of protein) taken from muscle protein.

CARBOHYDRATES

Carbohydrate is the preferred source of fuel for moderate- to high-intensity *aerobic* metabolism because it can be used more efficiently for ATP production than fat or protein. In fact, it is essential that carbohydrate be available if exercise is to continue for any sustained period of time.

The carbohydrate that is used during aerobic metabolism comes from both muscle glycogen stores and blood glucose. This is important, because although you cannot increase muscle glycogen levels during exercise, you can increase blood glucose levels through consumption of a carbohydrate drink or snack. In an average-size man, about 525 grams of glycogen are stored in the muscles with another 25 grams of glucose in the blood. The liver stores an additional 100 grams of glycogen, which can be broken down to glucose and released into the bloodstream to maintain blood glucose as it is being used by the tissues of the body. This is enough carbohydrate to support moderate-intensity exercise for about two hours.

FAT

Fat is the body's most concentrated fuel source. Unlike the carbohydrate stores, fat stores can fuel hours of exercise without running out. In fact, a 200-pound man with 15 percent body fat has about 130,000 calories of energy stored as fat. This is enough energy to run from Washington, D.C., to Miami.

Because the majority of fat is stored in adipose tissue, however, it is not readily available for fueling the muscles. Also ATP production is less efficient and therefore slower with fat than it is with carbohydrate. For this reason, fat can be used as a sole fuel source only during low-intensity exercise. Another important limitation on the use of fat as an energy source is the mandatory requirement for carbohydrate. In other words, "fat burns in a carbohydrate flame." Thus, when muscle glycogen is depleted, the ability of the muscles to use fat as an energy source is severely compromised.

PROTEIN

The use of protein for ATP production occurs when carbohydrate stores are low. During exercise, when the glycogen stores of the liver and muscles are starting to become depleted, muscle proteins are broken down into amino acids and are used as fuel. Most athletes do not realize the extent to which protein contributes to ATP production. In extended exercise, up to 15 percent of the muscle's energy needs are met by protein. Muscle protein breakdown during exercise results in muscle damage and soreness. However, you can minimize the use of protein for energy and its consequences with the proper nutrient supplementation, as you'll see in the next chapter.

REGULATORS OF ENERGY PRODUCTION

The metabolism of carbohydrate, fat, and protein in aerobic energy production is controlled in part by the endocrine system. Endocrine glands found throughout the body secrete hormones into the bloodstream. Hormones regulate many metabolic functions. They are classified according to function as catabolic (relating to breakdown) or anabolic (relating to buildup).

The major catabolic hormones are epinephrine (also known as adrenaline), norepinephrine (also known as noradrenaline), and cortisol. At the onset of exercise, these hormones are released and help initiate the breakdown of stored fuels. As exercise intensity or duration increases, or if there is a drop in blood glucose, the blood levels of these hormones will increase, thereby providing additional fuel for the muscle. The primary actions of epinephrine and norepinephrine are to increase the breakdown of fat and glycogen stored in the liver and muscle. Cortisol, on the other hand, stimulates the breakdown of fat and muscle protein. High levels of cortisol also suppress immune function. As you will see in Chapter 3, elevated levels of cortisol can dramatically slow muscle recovery after exercise.

The most important anabolic hormone is insulin. Insulin increases muscle glucose and amino acid transport and the synthesis of muscle glycogen. Insulin can also increase muscle blood flow. During exercise, insulin levels decline as the transport of glucose into the muscle and muscle blood flow are controlled by muscle contraction. However, after exercise, an increase in blood insulin levels is critical to the recovery process. It is vital to the replenishment of muscle glycogen, the repair of muscle tissue damaged during exercise, and the physiological adaptations that occur with training. Elevating insulin during exercise by supplementing with carbohydrate can also increase reliance on blood glucose as a fuel source and spare muscle glycogen.

CAUSES OF EXERCISE-RELATED FATIGUE

There are many causes of fatigue, but almost all of them are consequences of the muscles' attempt to generate the necessary energy for muscle contraction. The actual cause of fatigue in each individual case is specific to the type of exercise being performed. For the endurance athlete and those who play team sports, fatigue is usually the result of heat stress resulting from dehydration or the depletion of muscle glycogen.

Dehydration

Although the muscle machinery is extremely efficient in converting fuel to energy, it is not perfect. In general, about 60 percent of the energy released during exercise is wasted as heat rather than used to fuel muscle contractions. By comparison, a well-tuned engine is only about

30 percent efficient, which means 70 percent of the energy is lost as heat. In both cases, it is imperative that this excess heat be removed. As heat builds up, engine performance begins to decline. Even when the gas tank is full and the carburetor is delivering adequate amounts of fuel, the engine stops functioning if the cooling system fails. This is similar to what happens during exercise. When body temperature rises above a certain temperature, muscle contraction fails. For optimum exercise performance, body temperature must be controlled within fairly narrow limits.

The higher the intensity of exercise, the more heat is produced. Energy production from muscle contraction can theoretically increase the temperature of the body about 2°F every five minutes at high exercise intensities in a warm environment. Body temperature is normally 98.6°F. If it increases to 102.2°F, exercise performance is compromised. If it reaches 105.8°F, it can be life threatening and require medical attention.

There are several mechanisms that the body can use to maintain a stable temperature, one of which is direct transfer to the environment. For example, during running or cycling, excess body heat can be dissipated as cool air moves over the surface of the body. During swimming, excess body heat can be transferred to the cooler water. Direct transfer to the environment, however, is generally not an efficient means of dissipating heat. During intense exercise, the primary cooling mechanism is sweat evaporation, which accounts for about 80 percent of total heat loss.

To rapidly dissipate heat generated by the muscles, it must be transferred to the blood vessels surrounding the muscles and carried by the bloodstream to vessels just below the surface of the skin. As the skin temperature rises, sweat glands are activated and release sweat, which then evaporates, cooling both the skin and the blood just below. The cooled blood can then be returned to the muscles to help dissipate additional heat.

The need to move blood from the muscles to the skin to dissipate heat can put a strain on the heart and cardiovascular system because of the requirement to pump blood to the skin as well as to the working muscles. The warmer and more humid the environment, the greater the sweat rate and skin blood flow required to dissipate the heat generated by the muscles. As body water is lost, blood volume declines. This decline limits the capacity of the circulatory system to carry oxygen and nutrients to, and remove metabolic byproducts (such as lactic acid) as well as heat from, the exercising muscles. This results in a rise in body temperature, causing fatigue.

The effect of dehydration on the cardiovascular system is immediately evident. For each 1 percent loss in body weight due to sweating, heart rate increases five to eight beats per minute and the amount of blood pumped declines. When dehydration occurs in a hot environment, it has a more adverse effect on performance because direct transfer of heat to the environment is less effective, putting additional pressure on sweating to cool the body.

The loss of body fluid equal to as little as 2 percent body weight (approximately 3.5 pounds for a 175-pound athlete) can significantly reduce blood volume, putting stress on the cardiovascular system and limiting physical performance. As dehydration increases, performance continues to decrease (see Table 2.1). Reduction in performance can occur in the form of reduced stamina and deterioration of fine motor skills such as eye-hand coordination and mental alertness. When dehydration approaches 4 percent, athletes can experience heat cramps (cramps in skeletal muscles accompanied by profuse sweating) and heat exhaustion (dizziness, weakness, nausea, and possibly collapse). When dehydration approaches 6 percent, it can result in heatstroke. Symptoms of heatstroke are severe headache, cessation of sweating, a rapid rise in body temperature, collapse, and unconsciousness. Heatstroke is a life-threatening condition that requires immediate medical attention.

A consequence of sweating is the loss of electrolytes, including sodium, potassium, and chloride, which are necessary for many metabolic functions such as muscle contraction and nerve transmission. Generally, the composition of sodium and chloride in sweat is about one-third that found in blood. It is not uncommon for athletes to lose up to 9 pounds of fluid by sweating during an extended workout or long race. With such a fluid loss, the electrolyte losses would be roughly 5 to 6 percent of the body's total sodium and chloride content. Potassium losses would be significant, as well. Some of the symptoms resulting from sodium loss are reduced performance, dizziness, and fainting. Some of the symptoms resulting from potassium loss are nausea, diminished reflexes, fluctuation in heart rate, muscular fatigue, and weakness.

2.1. EFFECT OF INCREASING DEHYDRATION ON PHYSICAL PERFORMANCE

Body Water Loss	Effects
0.5%	Increased strain on the heart
1%	Reduced aerobic endurance
3%	Reduced muscular endurance
4%	Reduced muscle strength; reduced fine motor skills; heat cramps
5%	Heat exhaustion; cramping; fatigue; reduced mental capacity
6%	Physical exhaustion; heatstroke; coma

Muscle Glycogen Depletion

More than fifty years ago, researchers showed that the depletion of muscle glycogen was highly related to fatigue during prolonged endurance exercise and exercise of high intensity. The reason muscle glycogen is so important is that it is the only fuel that can be used by both the anaerobic and aerobic energy systems. As illustrated in Figure 2.4 on page 20, as exercise intensity increases, the rate at which muscle glycogen is used also increases. When you are exercising at 70 percent VO_2max, your muscle glycogen stores will last about two and a half hours. At 85 percent VO_2max, your glycogen stores will last only about thirty minutes.

During very intense and explosive movements lasting more than a few seconds, glycolysis is the only energy system that can generate ATP fast enough to meet the muscles' energy requirements for such activities. These types of activities cannot be sustained for long periods of time because of the rapid accumulation of lactic acid, the byproduct of glycolysis. As lactic acid accumulates, it inhibits the muscles' metabolic pathways, reducing ATP production and eventually causing fatigue. Exercise can continue if the intensity is reduced before a critical level of lactic acid accumulates. During exercise performed at a lower intensity that does not rely heavily on glycolysis for ATP production, the lactic acid previously produced can be removed by the liver and converted

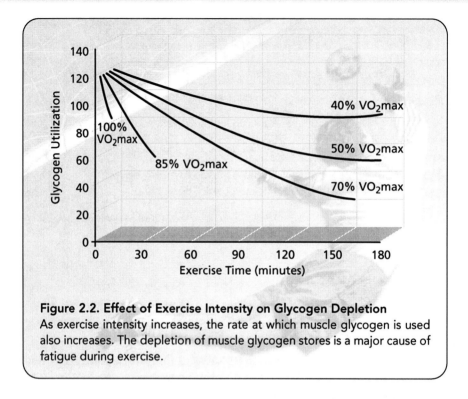

Figure 2.2. Effect of Exercise Intensity on Glycogen Depletion
As exercise intensity increases, the rate at which muscle glycogen is used also increases. The depletion of muscle glycogen stores is a major cause of fatigue during exercise.

into glucose. For example, a defenseman on a hockey team may produce a considerable amount of lactic acid when he's tightly guarding an opponent with the puck, but he will be able to recover (that is, the lactic acid can be converted to glucose) when the puck changes sides or when he is relieved by another player.

The exercise intensity above which lactic acid accumulates rapidly is referred to as the "lactate threshold." One's lactate (lactic acid) threshold is highly associated with one's ability to sustain relatively high levels of exercise intensity for extended periods.

When the exercise intensity allows for a prolonged effort such as running a 10,000-meter race, ATP is mainly produced by the aerobic energy system. Aerobic metabolism does not result in a significant accumulation of lactic acid, but the rate of ATP production is substantially less than can be produced anaerobically. The aerobic energy system relies predominately on fat and carbohydrate for fuel, but as the exercise intensity increases, the reliance on carbohydrate, particularly muscle glycogen, takes precedence. When muscle glycogen is depleted, only exercise of moderate intensity can be sustained, because fat and blood glucose cannot be burned with enough efficiency to support high-intensity activity. This is very evident to the marathon runner who has "hit the wall" at mile 20 or the cyclist who has "bonked" during the latter stages of a road race.

OTHER CONSEQUENCES OF EXERCISE

Every time you take your car for a drive, there are residual effects. The fuel supply decreases, carbon builds up around the pistons, and the wear on the engine parts increase. This is also the case for our bodies. Each time we exercise, our fuel supplies are reduced, waste builds up, and the wear on our body parts increases.

Muscle Damage

An unavoidable outcome of exercise is muscle damage. Some of this muscle damage is beneficial, since a mild breakdown of muscle protein stimulates the rebuilding process. Almost all aerobic athletes have at one time or another felt stiff or sore following their exercise bouts. In the short term, this can be due to the accumulation of lactic acid in the muscles, but lactic acid is removed from the muscles within sixty minutes and cannot account for residual muscle soreness that lasts for several days. This lasting soreness is due to muscle damage and inflammation.

There are three primary causes of muscle damage: mechanical, hormonal, and oxidative. The last two causes are directly related to the muscles' need for energy. It is important to understand how each of these factors contributes to muscle damage, because nutrient intervention within the Performance Zone can greatly reduce muscle damage, accelerating recovery between serious training sessions.

Initial damage occurs as a result of the physical forces acting on the muscles, which oppose muscle contraction. Muscle contractions place stress on the muscles, which can lead to tearing of the muscle fibers. Muscle injury triggers an acute inflammatory response, and within hours, specific cells migrate to the site of the damage and begin removing tissue debris. This process causes swelling, which can further damage muscle cell membranes. The acute inflammatory response does not peak for up to twenty-four hours, which is one reason why muscle soreness is often not felt until well after the exercise is completed.

The second cause of muscle damage is the catabolic hormone cortisol. Cortisol is released from the adrenal glands when blood glucose is low and during high-intensity exercise. The primary function of cortisol is to generate fuel for working muscles by stimulating the breakdown of protein for energy. The greater the protein breakdown, the greater the muscle damage.

The third cause of muscle damage is the formation of free radicals, which is also related to the need to generate energy. Free radicals are highly reactive molecules that are formed in the presence of oxygen. Normally, free radicals can be inactivated by natural antioxidants that exist in the body. However, during exercise, as oxygen consumption increases, there is a parallel increase in free-radical formation. The resulting flood of free radicals overwhelms the body's natural antioxidant mechanisms, damaging muscle protein, injuring cell membranes, and even deactivating key enzymes responsible for proper functioning of the immune system.

Suppression of the Immune System

Athletes who train hard day after day are more susceptible to colds and infections. Although this is commonly seen in professional and collegiate sports wherein travel schedules and high frequency of play tend to add stress to the life of the athlete, it is also seen in everyday athletes who simply train extremely hard. There are several reasons for the immunosuppressive effects of strenuous exercise. These include an increase in blood levels of cortisol and a decline in blood levels of the amino acid glutamine and glucose. Cortisol lowers the concentration and reduces the activities of many of the important infection-fighting immune cells. Although blood cortisol levels increase during strenuous exercise or when blood glucose declines, they also increase during periods of mental stress. Therefore, other stresses in an athlete's life (for example, lack of sleep and school/work demands) can exacerbate the immunosuppressive effects of hard training. Immune system suppression can last up to seventy-two hours following exercise.

Glutamine, the most prevalent amino acid found in muscle, is important in maintaining immune function. During strenuous exercise, muscle levels of glutamine are severely depleted. Studies have shown a causal relationship between the depletion of glutamine and an athlete's susceptibility to infection.

SUMMARY

ATP is the only source of energy that can drive muscle contraction, but there is only enough ATP stored in the muscles to support a maximal effort for a few seconds. Therefore, ATP must be continually replenished during exercise by other metabolic systems. During prolonged exercise, there are a number of metabolic, physiological, and hormonal changes that must occur if the ATP requirements are to be met. While essential, these changes also result in temporary adverse effects such as a loss of body water, reduced blood volume, a depletion of carbohydrate stores, muscle damage, and suppression of the immune system. The degree of these adverse effects is related to both the intensity and the duration of exercise. Moreover, these adverse effects can persist for long periods of time after exercise and, if not addressed, can slow recovery and exercise-training adaptations. Fortunately, as you will learn in Chapter 3, these adverse effects can be reduced by nutrient supplementation at the appropriate time, resulting in greater endurance and a faster recovery.

3.

Fueling Muscles Before and During Exercise

The need to control body temperature and to supply adequate amounts of ATP to working muscles during exercise results in a number of physiological and metabolic changes that can lead to a decline in performance and eventually fatigue. As discussed in this chapter, the severity of these changes can be reduced with appropriate nutrient supplementation.

PREPARING THE BODY FOR EXERCISE

For most athletes, their workout begins when they start stretching. However, by redefining when your workout begins, you can jump-start the refueling process. Nutrients and fluids consumed in the thirty-minute period prior to your exercise can deliver big benefits.

Because of the immediate and dramatic effects of dehydration on sports performance, we recommend that athletes consume 14–20 ounces of water or electrolyte solution thirty minutes before prolonged intense exercise in the heat. Consumption of fluids during this time will delay the development of dehydration, speed the onset of sweating, and cause a smaller rise in body temperature. Electrolyte solutions are preferred over pure water because the addition of electrolytes prevents the excretion of water through the kidneys. By consuming a drink with electrolytes, your body retains the fluid you need, thereby avoiding the frequent and annoying need to urinate during exercise or competition.

The consumption of carbohydrate in the hour before exercise can help increase glycogen stores and raise blood glucose and insulin levels. But the practice of consuming carbohydrate in the hour prior to exercise has proven to be controversial. Initial research suggested that this practice would elevate blood insulin levels prior to exercise, which would cause excessive blood glucose and muscle glycogen utilization and result in premature fatigue. This finding has not been substantiated by current research. In fact, many studies have found that supplementing with certain nutrients prior to exercise can actually improve aerobic performance, particularly if sufficient carbohydrate is consumed. Consuming 6 ounces of an easily digestible carbohydrate plus 18–20 ounces of water about thirty minutes prior to exercise will help jump-start the fueling process. However, a more effective approach is to consume 18–20 ounces of a carbohydrate/protein sports drink containing 6 to 8 percent carbohydrate and 1.5 to 2 percent protein. This sports drink can also be used as your hydration drink at the start of exercise and periodically during exercise. Pre-exercise consumption of a carbohydrate/protein sports drink will initiate the absorption of needed carbohydrate and amino acids at the onset of exercise, reducing use of the body's own fuel stores. It will also provide fluid to support heat dissipation. This will help increase endurance during exercise and recovery post-exercise.

DURING EXERCISE

The importance of proper nutrition during exercise cannot be overstated. It can prevent overheating, increase endurance, help maintain fine motor skills, limit tissue damage, and even accelerate muscle recovery. Every serious athlete must have a nutritional program for training and competition. The major goals for fueling muscles during exercise are:

➤ Prevent dehydration and electrolyte loss.

➤ Maintain carbohydrate availability and spare muscle glycogen.

➤ Limit muscle damage.

➤ Limit suppression of the immune system.

➤ Set the stage for a faster recovery following your workout.

Prevent Dehydration and Electrolyte Loss

Once exercise starts, you should try to fully replace fluid losses that occur. The amount of fluid lost during exercise by sweating depends on a number of factors, but the most important are exercise intensity, ambient temperature, and individual sweat rates. Table 3.1 shows the amount of fluid lost per hour of exercise based on low, moderate, and high sweat rates when exercising at a moderate intensity (70 percent VO_2max) in different ambient temperatures.

3.1. AVERAGE SWEAT RATE AT MODERATE EXERCISE INTENSITY* FOR DIFFERENT TEMPERATURES

Temperature	Sweat Rate (ounces per hour)		
	Low	Moderate	High
40°F	12	17	35
55°F	15	22	31
70°F	22	27	47
90°F	31	37	75

*70 percent VO_2max

You can estimate your own standard rate of sweat loss by weighing yourself immediately before and after a typical workout and calculating the difference. For example, suppose you lose 2 pounds during a two-hour workout. Two pounds is equivalent to 32 ounces of water. You should plan to replace about 32 ounces of water during this workout. This can be accomplished by consuming 4 ounces every fifteen minutes. In Chapter 6, we'll show you an easy way to calculate your fluid losses during exercise.

Table 3.1 also illustrates that under extreme environmental conditions, sweat rate can exceed the maximum rate of fluid absorption in the digestive tract (between 34 and 40 ounces per hour). As a general rule, when sweat rates are high, you should try to consume as much fluid as you can tolerate during workouts and competitions. The key is to develop a plan that calls for drinking whenever time permits. You should also try to drink small amounts of fluid frequently rather than larger amounts only occasionally. For example, drink every ten to fifteen minutes during a marathon. You cannot depend on your thirst mechanisms to tell you when and how much to drink. Athletes left to voluntarily drink during exercise will replace only 30 to 50 percent of the fluid lost.

Because sweat is composed chiefly of water and electrolytes, it is important for several reasons to also replace the electrolytes that are lost through sweating. First, electrolytes help maintain your body's fluid balance. Second, including electrolytes in your sports drink will stimulate your thirst mechanisms. Whereas drinking pure water to quench your thirst quickly reduces the drive to drink, the addition of electrolytes maintains this drive, resulting in a more adequate fluid consumption. Third, electrolyte replacement helps maintain blood volume. Finally, electrolyte replacement prevents hyponatremia, a deficiency of sodium in the blood.

Hyponatremia occurs when blood volume increases at the same time electrolyte content decreases. Symptoms include bloating, headaches, nausea, vomiting, muscle weakness, cramping, and seizures. Acute hyponatremia has a mortality rate of about 50 percent. Although hyponatremia occurs infrequently, it must be taken seriously.

Sodium and chloride are the primary electrolytes found in sweat, but sweat also contains significant amounts of potassium and some magnesium. Most sports drinks are formulated to provide the proper ratio of electrolytes to adequately replace those lost in sweat.

Maintain Carbohydrate Availability and Spare Muscle Glycogen

The importance of maintaining carbohydrate stores during exercise has been shown in many studies. For example, in a study conducted at the University of Texas at Austin, well-trained cyclists exercised at a moderate to high aerobic intensity to exhaustion with or without carbohydrate supplementation. In the absence of supplementation, fatigue occurred at three hours of exercise and was preceded by a decline in blood glucose. When the cyclists received carbohydrate supplementation, which prevented the decline in blood glucose, they were able to exercise for four hours before becoming fatigued.

Similar results were seen involving high-intensity intermittent exercise. After three hours of high-intensity intermittent exercise, cyclists who received a carbohydrate supplement were able to exercise at 80 percent VO_2max for thirty-three minutes versus two minutes for cyclists who received flavored water. The improvement with the carbohydrate supplement was due to a sparing of muscle glycogen.

Participants in team sports also benefit from carbohydrate supplementation. Soccer players were found to run more and perform better during a soccer match, particularly during the second half, when they received carbohydrate supplementation. Even motor skills appear to be better maintained during the later stages of athletic contests. For example, when supplemented with carbohydrate versus a placebo (flavored water), tennis players are more accurate with their shots and make fewer errors during the final sets of a tennis match.

The greatest performance benefits have been found when 50–70 grams of carbohydrate are consumed per hour of exercise. This amount reflects the body's maximum rate of carbohydrate absorption. When greater amounts are consumed, stomach cramping and other gastrointestinal problems often result.

Sports drinks that are formulated to address fluid, electrolyte, and carbohydrate needs should contain 1.75–2.4 grams of carbohydrate per ounce of water (a 6 to 8 percent solution). When the carbohydrate concentration exceeds 10 percent, it slows the movement of fluid into the circulatory system, the result of which is compromised regulation of body temperature during exercise.

TIMING OF CARBOHYDRATE CONSUMPTION

In general, glycogen stores are sufficient for a minimum of forty-five to sixty minutes of moderate-intensity exercise (75 percent VO_2max). So supplements do not necessarily have to be consumed immediately upon the start of exercise. There, is however, a strong rationale for starting supplementation immediately. In doing so, your muscles begin using blood glucose as a source of energy, thereby sparing muscle glycogen stores. And of course, if fluid replacement is a concern because of high temperatures, you'll need to begin consuming fluids immediately.

Under hot, humid conditions, consuming 7 ounces of a 7 percent carbohydrate solution every fifteen minutes provides 54 grams of carbohydrate and 27 ounces of fluid per hour. Starting supplementation early and continuing throughout exercise is also advisable when the exercise intensity will vary considerably or when activity will be interrupted by periodic rest periods, such as during an ice-hockey game. This increases the reliance on blood glucose and spares muscle glycogen during the periods of low activity.

TYPES OF CARBOHYDRATE

The effects of solid and liquid carbohydrate supplements are similar when heat stress is not a factor. However, liquid carbohydrate supplements are more beneficial than solid carbohydrates when exercising in a warm environment. The ideal type of carbohydrate is high glycemic. The glycemic index is a method of categorizing foods by their effect on blood glucose levels. A low-glycemic food produces a mild sustained increase in blood glucose levels whereas a high-glycemic food produces a larger rapid increase in blood glucose. High-glycemic carbohydrates such as glucose, maltodextrin, and sucrose when taken alone or in combination have the most beneficial and also similar effects on athletic performance. The sugars fructose and galactose have a lower glycemic index. They should not be used in high concentration or as the sole carbohydrate in a sports drink. Fructose is absorbed from the intestines half as fast as glucose, and produces a lower blood glucose and insulin response. Consuming large amounts of fructose during exercise can result in an upset stomach, diarrhea, and inadequate rate of glucose availability. Galactose may also increase the use of muscle glycogen for energy. Therefore, it is recommended that glucose, sucrose, or maltodextrin comprise the majority of carbohydrate in a sports drink.

ADDITION OF PROTEIN

Carbohydrate/electrolyte sports drinks have been the standard for almost thirty-five years. But this is changing. A number of newer studies have established the benefits of adding protein to a sports drink. Researchers recently reported that a drink containing carbohydrate and protein in a 4:1 ratio improved endurance 57 percent compared with water and 24 percent compared with a carbohydrate drink during high-intensity cycling. This is illustrated in Figure 3.1. The improvement in endurance was thought to be due to a sparing of muscle glycogen and possibly to the preferential use of the ingested protein rather than muscle protein as an energy source.

Similar results were recently demonstrated in a study conducted at James Madison University in which cyclists received a carbohydrate/protein drink or carbohydrate supplement during moderate-intensity exercise. The cyclists receiving the carbohydrate/protein drink were able to exercise almost 30 percent longer than when they were given a carbohydrate supplement.

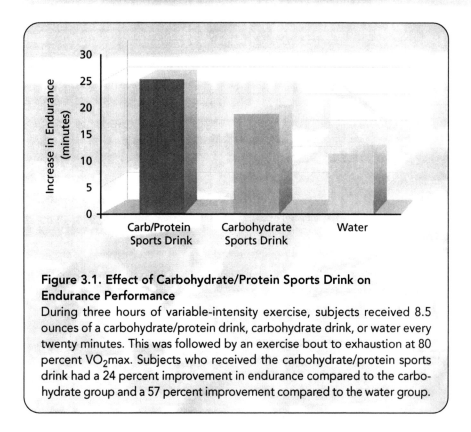

Figure 3.1. Effect of Carbohydrate/Protein Sports Drink on Endurance Performance
During three hours of variable-intensity exercise, subjects received 8.5 ounces of a carbohydrate/protein drink, carbohydrate drink, or water every twenty minutes. This was followed by an exercise bout to exhaustion at 80 percent VO$_2$max. Subjects who received the carbohydrate/protein sports drink had a 24 percent improvement in endurance compared to the carbohydrate group and a 57 percent improvement compared to the water group.

Limit Muscle Damage

Nutrient intervention can help limit muscle damage during exercise, but it must be designed to focus on the different causes. Nutrient intervention has no effect on damage caused by physical forces, but it can impact damage caused by increased levels of cortisol and free radicals. Carbohydrate supplementation during exercise can reduce blood levels of cortisol, thereby reducing muscle tissue breakdown and limiting overall muscle damage.

Muscle damage resulting from free radicals can also be limited by supplementing with antioxidants such as vitamins E and C during exercise. Although there doesn't appear to be a performance benefit from antioxidant supplementation, researchers have observed that supplementation with vitamins E and C decreased markers of muscle damage twenty-four hours after a marathon.

The addition of protein to a carbohydrate supplement also appears to reduce muscle damage. While investigating the benefits of carbohydrate/protein supplementation on endurance performance, researchers at James Madison University measured postexercise blood levels of creatine phosphokinase (CPK), a marker of muscle damage. As illustrated in Figure 3.2, the subjects who received the carbohydrate/protein supplement had CPK levels 83 percent lower than those subjects who received the carbohydrate supplement, indicating significantly less muscle damage during exercise.

Although the exact mechanism by which protein reduces muscle damage remains undetermined, two possibilities have been suggested: 1) The body may favor the protein in sports drinks over muscle protein for energy production during extended exercise, resulting in less damage to the muscles, and 2) The protein may raise amino acid levels in the blood. Elevated levels of amino acids have been shown to reduce the breakdown of muscle protein.

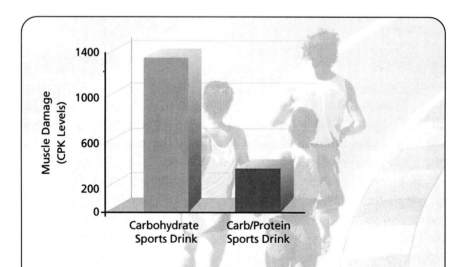

Figure 3.2. Effect of Carbohydrate/Protein Supplementation on Muscle Damage
Levels of CPK, a marker of muscle damage, were measured fifteen hours after subjects completed an endurance ride during which they received either a carbohydrate/protein supplement or a carbohydrate supplement. CPK levels in subjects who received the carbohydrate/protein supplement were 83 percent lower than they were in subjects who received carbohydrate only.

Limit Suppression of the Immune System

During intense aerobic training, cortisol levels can increase fivefold. Given the close relationship between high cortisol levels and immune system suppression, and the fact that carbohydrate supplementation inhibits cortisol release, it seems logical that carbohydrate supplementation would limit the suppressive effects of exercise on the immune system. In fact, this has been confirmed by several studies from Appalachian State University. Athletes who fail to supplement with nutrients during their workouts are more likely to experience the immunosuppressive effects of cortisol, which include a temporary weakening of the body's major infection-fighting mechanisms.

Set the Stage for a Faster Recovery Following Your Workout

Training hard without appropriate nutrient intervention results in a prolonged recovery, a lower-quality training program, and ultimately a weaker training response. Although you cannot completely eliminate the depletion of energy stores or avoid muscle damage during strenuous training sessions, you can minimize these effects and set the stage for a faster recovery by employing the appropriate nutrient intervention.

Because there is increased muscle breakdown during exercise, consuming protein in a supplement during exercise will allow your muscles to use the supplemental protein for their energy needs and spare muscle protein. This results in less muscle damage. The same principle holds true with regard to muscle glycogen. Maintaining blood glucose levels by consuming carbohydrate during exercise results in less depletion of glycogen stores.

Findings from James Madison University reinforce the concept that appropriate nutrient intervention during exercise will speed recovery. After demonstrating the beneficial effects of carbohydrate/protein supplementation on endurance performance in cyclists, researchers asked subjects to return after a fifteen-hour recovery period. Upon returning, the subjects performed a ride to exhaustion at 85 percent of their VO_2max. Subjects who received the carbohydrate/protein drink during the initial performance ride the day before were able to ride almost 40 percent longer than those subjects who had received the carbohydrate-only drink. (See Figure 3.3 on page 34.) These results are a strong testimony to the positive influence that appropriate supplementation during exercise can have on an athlete's subsequent exercise performance.

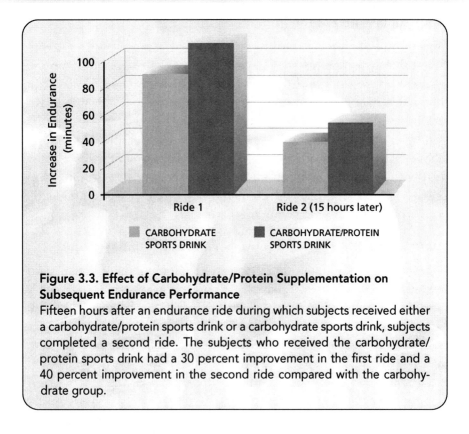

Figure 3.3. Effect of Carbohydrate/Protein Supplementation on Subsequent Endurance Performance
Fifteen hours after an endurance ride during which subjects received either a carbohydrate/protein sports drink or a carbohydrate sports drink, subjects completed a second ride. The subjects who received the carbohydrate/protein sports drink had a 30 percent improvement in the first ride and a 40 percent improvement in the second ride compared with the carbohydrate group.

GUIDELINES FOR EXERCISE NUTRITION

Nutrient supplementation beginning thirty minutes prior to starting your workout and continuing every fifteen to twenty minutes during the workout will not only improve your athletic performance but also lay the groundwork for a faster recovery following your workout. The ideal sports drink to consume during exercise should be composed of the ingredients listed in Table 3.2. Each of these ingredients is discussed below.

Water and Electrolytes

If exercise is to exceed sixty minutes and will take place under environmental conditions that will challenge the body's ability to maintain a stable temperature, we recommend that you consume 14–20 ounces of fluid, preferably a sports drink that contains electrolytes among other nutrients, thirty minutes prior to exercise.

During exercise, try to continually replace fluid lost as sweat by drinking at ten- to fifteen-minute intervals. Specific details for setting up your own schedule will be discussed in Chapter 6. In addition to water, sodium and potassium lost in sweat can also negatively impact performance. When replacing fluid loss, make sure electrolytes are included in your beverage.

Carbohydrate

Most sports drinks contain carbohydrate in the right concentration (6 to 8 percent) as well as electrolytes. As you've learned, carbohydrate is an essential fuel source during aerobic exercise. When your carbohydrate stores are depleted, your muscles will become fatigued and you will have to stop exercising or significantly reduce your exercise intensity. Consume 50–70 grams of carbohydrate per hour of exercise. Consuming 7 ounces of a 7 percent carbohydrate drink every fifteen minutes during exercise will provide 27 ounces of fluid and 54 grams of carbohydrate.

Protein

The addition of protein to a carbohydrate sports drink in amounts sufficient for a rate of consumption of 8–15 grams per hour can help improve

3.2. IDEAL NUTRIENT COMPOSITION FOR A SPORTS DRINK DURING EXERCISE

Nutrient Objectives	Ideal Composition (per 12 oz water)
• Replace fluids and electrolytes • Preserve muscle glycogen	High-glycemic carbohydrates, such as glucose, sucrose, and maltodextrin: 20–26 g
• Maintain blood glucose levels	Whey protein: 5–6 g
• Minimize cortisol increases	Vitamin C: 30–120 mg
• Set the stage for a faster recovery	Vitamin E: 20–60 IU
	Sodium: 100–250 mg
	Potassium: 60–120 mg
	Magnesium: 60–120 mg

endurance performance, reduce muscle protein degradation, and speed postexercise recovery. The protein of choice is whey because it is rapidly absorbed and contains all of the essential amino acids as well as a high percentage of leucine and glutamine, two amino acids that the body uses extensively during sustained exercise. For aerobic athletes, the ideal ratio of carbohydrate to protein is 4 grams of carbohydrate to 1 gram of protein. This formulation is highly digestible, does not interfere with hydration, and is proven to provide significant endurance and recovery benefits.

Vitamins

It may also be helpful to include the antioxidants vitamins C and E in your sports drink. There doesn't appear to be a performance benefit from antioxidant supplementation, but there is evidence that these vitamins may help limit muscle damage during prolonged exercise.

SUMMARY

Although fluid is the most important nutrient during exercise, the addition of carbohydrate and protein has been shown in many clinical studies to significantly improve athletic performance. The addition of carbohydrate can delay fatigue, inhibit cortisol release, and even help maintain immune function. The new generation of sports drink that contain carbohydrate and protein in a 4:1 ratio appear to further improve endurance, reduce muscle damage, and set the stage for a faster recovery after exercise.

Nutrition Focus

FUELING THE YOUNG ATHLETE
by Jeffrey Stout, Ph.D.

The young athlete in your family has a competition this morning. She starts the day with a breakfast of cereal and milk and washes it down with a glass of orange juice. That's the last time she has anything to eat or drink until halftime, when she has some water or a sports drink. Afterward, the players celebrate the game's completion (and possibly their victory) with a snack, such as potato chips and soda.

Well, the breakfast wasn't bad, but everything your young athlete did or didn't do in terms of in-game and postgame nutrition decreased her ability to play well, increased the likelihood of injuries, and greatly limited her ability to recover from the physical stresses of the game. Don't feel bad. Few parents think beyond breakfast when it comes to sports nutrition, and coaches, particularly at the youth level, are often too busy to worry about nutrition during the game.

The nutrition young athletes take in before, during, and after games or practices is critical to their performance. There are three factors you should consider when refueling a young athlete. Just think of the three Rs: **R**ehydrate, **R**eplenish, **R**ecover.

REHYDRATE

Dehydration, particularly among young athletes, is associated with heat-related injuries. Heatstroke is the second leading cause of death among high school athletes. Even in professional sports with well-trained doctors and coaches, athletes routinely fall ill due to heat exhaustion. In young athletes, however, the risks are even greater. There are a number of reasons for this. Young athletes sweat at a lower rate. Sweating is the primary mechanism for keeping body temperature cool. As a result, young athletes tolerate temperature extremes less efficiently than adults. They get hotter during exercise. For all of these reasons, fluid replenishment, which increases sweat rate, is the number-one objective of exercise nutrition for the young athlete.

It is also important to keep in mind that using thirst as a cue to drink is not a reliable way to prevent dehydration. By the time we are thirsty, we have already entered the first stage of dehydration. A 2 percent reduction in body weight from fluid loss can lead to a significant decline in muscle strength and endurance and an increase in fatigue. That's only 2 pounds for a 100-pound athlete.

Rehydrating the young athlete must begin during competition and training. The young athlete should drink 3–4 ounces of water or sports drink every ten to fifteen minutes. For teens, the requirement increases to 4–8 ounces every fifteen minutes. After exercise, the young athlete should drink 20 ounces of water or preferably a sports drink for every pound of weight loss.

REPLENISH

Glycogen is the major fuel used to generate muscle energy. During extended exercise, such as a soccer game, muscle glycogen stores are depleted. Studies have shown that when this occurs, the body becomes fatigued, and there is a strong link between muscle fatigue and injuries. Consuming a sports drink with carbohydrate or perhaps one of the newer protein-containing sports drinks not only will provide your child with the fluid his or her body needs, but will also delay the depletion of muscle glycogen. The carbohydrate/protein drinks can also help your child recover faster, which is particularly important in tournaments when playing two or three contests per day is not uncommon.

RECOVER

The forty-five-minute interval immediately following a game or practice is critical if you want your child to recover rapidly and play at his or her best the next time. Snacks like potato chips and soda couldn't be worse. Carbonation in a soda makes athletes feel fuller faster so they drink less, which means they may not fully replenish the fluids lost during the game. Potato chips, candy, and the like are high in fat, which hampers the ability of the muscles to initiate repair processes and replenish muscle glycogen. Ideally, the post-practice or postgame meal should be high in carbohydrate (0.4–0.8 grams per pound of body weight) with some protein (0.1–0.2 grams per pound of body weight) within fifteen to thirty minutes of completing exercise.

There are few other factors that can match the potential of sports nutrition to enhance the play of your child or the child you coach. With a little knowledge and effort, you can fuel your young athletes to play better, safer, and longer.

NUTRITION GUIDELINES FOR YOUNG ATHLETES

	Good Choices	Bad Choices
Before Practice and Games	High-fiber breakfast cereal, sandwich, fruit, energy bar, sports drink, water	Eggs, whole milk, beans, soda, snack chips
During Practice and Games	Sports drink with protein	Fruit juice, any solid food
After Practice and Games	Sports drink with protein, fruit, energy bar	Snack chips, fast food, soda

Jeffrey Stout, Ph.D., is coauthor of *Fit Kids for Life: A Parent's Guide to Optimal Nutrition and Training for Young Athletes* (Basic Health Publications, 2004).

4.

Muscle Recovery
After Exercise

All of the body's important recovery and adaptive processes require specific nutrients to proceed optimally. For this reason, the period immediately following exercise is the most important in an athlete's day, from a nutritional perspective. Failure to consume adequate amounts of the right nutrients in a timely manner after exercise will compromise your recovery in a number of ways. Conversely, optimizing your postexercise nutrition will carry a wide range of benefits, from reduced muscle soreness to better performance in tomorrow's exercise.

The car engine analogy that we used previously to describe the functions and needs of muscles during exercise no longer applies after exercise. When a car engine is turned off, the damage to moving parts also ceases. This is not the case with your muscles. The metabolic processes set off during exercise continue to damage the muscles even after you stop exercising. This is why muscle soreness is often not felt until twenty-four hours after an exercise bout.

In the absence of the right combination of nutrients, the body machinery necessary for rebuilding and replenishing energy stores and repairing damaged muscle is overwhelmed. Yet most athletes neglect to consume nutrients postexercise. Many choose water, which certainly helps deal with dehydration. Others may select a conventional carbohydrate/electrolyte sports drink, which is certainly superior to water. But neither is optimal.

There are two important principles of recovery nutrition. The first is that recovery from exercise is time-dependent. In other words, there is only a brief period of time in which you can maximally activate the muscle cells' anabolic (rebuilding) processes. The other principle is that

optimum activation of the rebuilding process depends on the types of
nutrients you consume postexercise.

The Metabolic Window

Following exercise, there is a window of metabolic opportunity that
can make a major impact in your overall training program, if properly
exploited. As shown in Figure 4.1, the muscle cells' potential to initiate
rebuilding and replenishment peaks about fifteen minutes after exercise
and declines by as much as 40 percent within sixty minutes. This window of opportunity has a major effect on most of the muscle cells' anabolic processes, including glycogen storage and protein synthesis.

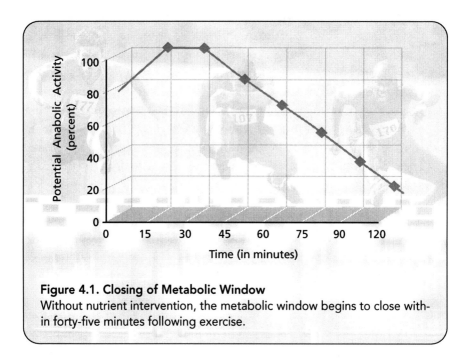

Figure 4.1. Closing of Metabolic Window
Without nutrient intervention, the metabolic window begins to close within forty-five minutes following exercise.

The transport of glucose into the muscle, which precedes glycogen
synthesis within the muscle, is three to four times faster when supplementation is taken immediately after exercise versus three hours later. In
fact, carbohydrate supplementation immediately after exercise results in
twice as much muscle glycogen storage as the same carbohydrate supplement consumed two hours later.

Insulin: The Master Rebuilding Hormone

Because of its association with carbohydrate, insulin has a negative image. Many people think that insulin is a "bad" hormone because it is linked with diabetes. But insulin does not cause diabetes. To the contrary, diabetes is a disease of insulin deficiency or resistance. For the athlete, insulin is the most important anabolic hormone in the body, controlling almost every major muscle cell activity and serving four important functions:

1. Insulin stimulates glucose transport and glycogen synthesis.

This is the most well known of insulin's effects. During exercise, glucose must be transported from the blood into the muscles, where it can be converted into energy. Insulin serves an important function here since the release of insulin stimulates the transport of glucose into the muscles.

Following exercise, the muscle machinery, in the presence of carbohydrate, begins the process of replenishing depleted glycogen stores. Insulin plays a major role in replenishing muscle glycogen stores by increasing the transport of glucose into the blood and by stimulating the enzymes responsible for manufacturing muscle glycogen.

2. Insulin suppresses cortisol.

For any athlete, cortisol is the enemy. Cortisol is a powerful catabolic hormone that causes the breakdown of protein. When cortisol levels are high, there is increased protein breakdown, which means that it takes longer for the muscles to fully recover following strenuous exercise. However, insulin has been shown to suppress the postexercise rise in cortisol levels.

3. Insulin increases net protein balance.

No other anabolic hormone has as significant an effect on protein synthesis as insulin. Insulin increases protein synthesis three ways. First, it increases the transport of amino acids (the building blocks of protein) into the muscles by as much as 50 percent. Second, insulin stimulates the enzymes necessary for protein synthesis by as much as 67 percent. And third, insulin reduces muscle protein degradation.

4. Insulin increases muscle blood flow.

During exercise, blood flow to working muscles can increase more than twentyfold. After exercise, however, muscle blood flow decreases to normal levels. Studies have shown that insulin can increase muscle blood flow preferentially by over 100 percent, resulting in faster removal of metabolic wastes, such as lactic acid and carbon dioxide, and a faster delivery of nutrients.

In the postexercise period, nutrient intervention can also profoundly affect protein metabolism. Researchers at Vanderbilt University observed that carbohydrate/protein supplementation immediately after exercise resulted in protein synthesis rates three times higher than when athletes received the same supplement three hours later. Additionally, protein breakdown was lower, and the all-important net protein balance (protein synthesis minus protein breakdown) increased significantly (that is, protein was being synthesized faster than it was being broken down). When the supplement was received three hours later, there was actually a net protein loss (protein was being broken down faster than it was being synthesized). These results have enormous implications for the aerobic athlete since the structural elements of the muscles as well as the enzymes responsible for generating energy and building and repairing the muscles are all composed of protein.

What Controls the Metabolic Window

The metabolic window is controlled by the actions of insulin, the anabolic regulator of the muscle cells. In the immediate postexercise period, muscle cells are exquisitely sensitive to the effect of insulin. To take full advantage of insulin's anabolic actions, the right combination of nutrients must be consumed while the muscles are insulin sensitive. However, the muscles rapidly lose their insulin sensitivity. It is greatly reduced after one hour of recovery, and after two hours, the muscles not only lose their sensitivity to insulin but actually become insulin resistant. Once insulin resistance develops, it can continue for up to sixteen hours after exercise. As shown in Figure 4.2, by delaying nutrient supplementation after exercise, almost every single important anabolic activity is decreased.

All is not lost, however. You can reverse this downward spiral toward muscle breakdown. But you are going to have to change your behavior. Following a hard workout, most athletes are simply not hungry right away. They may consume water or even a sports drink, but this is not enough. Flipping on the "anabolic switch" to generate a complete and speedy recovery requires a total nutritional approach.

SUMMARY

Nutritionally speaking, the period following exercise is the most important in an athlete's day. In the forty-five minutes after exercise, the mus-

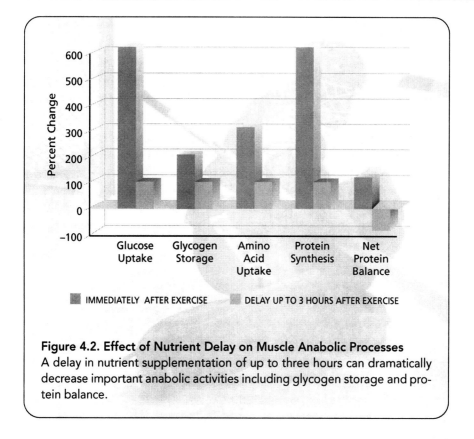

Figure 4.2. Effect of Nutrient Delay on Muscle Anabolic Processes
A delay in nutrient supplementation of up to three hours can dramatically decrease important anabolic activities including glycogen storage and protein balance.

cles' metabolic machinery is primed to rebuild and repair muscle tissue and replenish muscle energy stores. All that is needed is for the right combination of nutrients to be provided. The key to this metabolic window of opportunity is insulin, the muscle cells' most important anabolic regulator. In the immediate postexercise period, the muscle cells are extremely sensitive to the anabolic actions of insulin. The metabolic window is open only for a short period of time. Almost every important rebuilding process is significantly reduced if nutrient intervention following exercise is delayed more than forty-five minutes.

Nutrition Focus

FUELING THE FEMALE ATHLETE

by Kim Brown, M.S., R.D.

Since the passage of Title IX—the law that expanded opportunities for females in sports—more than thirty years ago, the number of females participating in various sport activities has skyrocketed. For example, it was recently reported that female finishers outnumbered male finishers for the first time at a major marathon of more than 20,000 runners. Such milestones are cause for celebration. However, in order to truly embrace the obvious benefits of sport participation, it is essential that athletes and coaches alike understand the unique nutritional demands that face the female gender during fitness training.

ENERGY INTAKE

Perhaps the most important nutritional consideration for females engaged in sport activity is an increased need for energy in the form of carbohydrate, fat, and protein to help fuel the working body. Inadequate caloric intake is a major problem among female athletes, who tend to be much more concerned about their weight than male athletes. The sad irony is that female athletes are far more likely to achieve the optimal body composition by increasing their intake of the appropriate nutrients than by enforcing unhealthy dietary restrictions. They will also perform much better in practice and competition if they avoid under-fueling their bodies. Avoiding this mistake will enhance the fitness benefits of the exercise.

Just like a car that stalls when it runs out of gas, the female athlete who doesn't consume adequate calories to support training will constantly battle fatigue during workouts and will also be more vulnerable to muscle injuries. In order to support daily training demands, female athletes who train at least an hour a day should aim to consume approximately nineteen to twenty plus calories per pound of lean body weight, with 55 to 60 percent of those calories being derived from carbohydrates (fruits, vegetables, and/or whole grains), 15 to 20 percent protein (cottage cheese, eggs, chicken, fish, beef, and/or soy), and 20 to 25 percent fat (olives, avocado, nuts, and/or seeds).

Additional calories are warranted when training exceeds ninety minutes. Perhaps the most convenient method of replenishing lost fluids, electrolytes, and carbohydrate during prolonged sport activity is through a sports drink containing these nutrients. Recent research also suggests that the addition of protein to a sports drink can delay fatigue and speed recovery even more than a carbohydrate/electrolyte mixture. See Chapter 6 for guidelines to determine the specific amounts of nutrients needed during and after exercise.

FLUID INTAKE

It is estimated that two out of every three female athletes walk around chronically dehydrated, which is a definite cause for concern since dehydration is the number-one dietary contributing factor to poor performance. On the flipside, some female athletes drink excessive amounts of water throughout the day, which can potentially be deadly. Female athletes should aim to consume half their body weight (in pounds) in fluid ounces each day, not including caffeinated beverages. For example, a 130-pound woman would aim to consume 65 ounces of water on a daily basis. An additional 4–8 ounces of fluid should be consumed every fifteen minutes during training. During exercise bouts lasting longer than sixty minutes, a sports drink that contains electrolytes is preferable.

MICRONUTRIENT INTAKE

The micronutrients calcium and iron are often lacking in the female athlete's diet, especially when energy intake is suboptimal. Poor eating habits combined with loss of iron in blood through menstruation puts the female athlete at risk for anemia, a condition marked by extreme fatigue and diminished performance. To improve iron intake, the female athlete should include more animal protein such as beef in her diet. For vegetarians, plant sources of iron such as whole grains, fortified cereals, and legumes should be combined with foods rich in vitamin C (such as oranges) to aid iron absorption.

Another common mineral deficiency among female athletes is calcium deficiency. Female athletes who are too caught up in the desire to lose weight often reduce their intake of calcium-rich dairy foods such as milk. At the same time, high levels of training can cause body-fat levels in some female athletes to fall so low that their production of estrogen decreases, ultimately preventing calcium from being diverted from the bloodstream to the bones, which increases the risk of stress fractures and osteoporosis. To boost calcium intake to the commonly recommended 800–1,200 milligrams per day, female athletes should aim to consume three to four servings of dairy per day. (One serving of dairy is equivalent to 1 cup of milk, 1 cup of yogurt, $1/2$ cup of part-skim ricotta cheese, or 1 piece of string cheese.)

Kim Brown, M.S., R.D., is a registered dietitian and competitive endurance athlete. She is also the nutrition columnist for *Triathlete* magazine.

5.
Fueling Muscles After Exercise

R esearch has clearly demonstrated the importance of taking advantage of the increased muscle insulin sensitivity that occurs immediately following exercise. For the athlete, it is really the metabolic window of opportunity. If you take advantage of it, you will be rewarded with faster recovery and a stronger workout the next time out. If you don't take advantage of it today, there is always tomorrow's workout. But remember, the muscle adaptations that lead to better sports performance are a result of a consistent exercise (and nutrition) routine. This means exploiting the metabolic window after every workout.

The major goals for nutrient supplementation during the recovery period are:

➤ Shift the metabolic machinery into an anabolic (muscle-building) state from a catabolic (muscle-depleting) state.

➤ Replenish muscle glycogen stores.

➤ Initiate tissue repair and set the stage for muscle growth.

➤ Reduce muscle damage and support the immune system.

➤ Start the replenishment of fluid and electrolytes.

Shift the Metabolic Machinery into a Muscle-Building State from a Muscle-Depleting State

Following exercise, the muscle machinery is in a catabolic mode, which means the breakdown of key muscle nutrients continues even though activity has ceased. However, you have the opportunity to "flip the anabolic switch" so that instead of breaking down muscle protein and nutrients, you can actually begin to rebuild the muscle, thereby initiating a much faster recovery. Insulin is the key.

Almost forty years ago, researchers noted that when protein was added to carbohydrate, it provided a strong stimulus for insulin release. Based on this observation, more recent studies have shown that a carbohydrate/protein combination is more effective than both carbohydrate alone and protein alone in stimulating insulin release. The stimulation of insulin release is the critical first step in muscle recovery, and this must be done immediately after the cessation of exercise if you are to take full advantage of the muscle's increased sensitivity to insulin.

Once the blood insulin level is increased in the presence of the right nutrients, insulin orchestrates multiple metabolic reactions critical for the repair and rebuilding of muscle cells.

Replenish Muscle Glycogen Stores

For the aerobic athlete, replenishing muscle glycogen stores is the most critical first step of muscle recovery. Depending on the exercise intensity and duration, muscle glycogen stores can be severely depleted following aerobic exercise. According to traditional thinking, all athletes need to do in order to stimulate muscle glycogen storage is to consume a carbohydrate drink. This approach, however, has limitations. Consuming carbohydrate will increase muscle glycogen storage to a point, but then the effect begins to plateau.

When protein is added to a carbohydrate supplement, the increase in blood insulin is greater than that produced by carbohydrate or protein alone. This translates into faster glycogen synthesis. In one study, a carbohydrate/protein supplement was found to be 38 percent more efficient in restoring muscle glycogen than a carbohydrate supplement and almost four times more efficient than a protein supplement.

Maximizing the rate of glycogen replenishment is especially important when exercise is frequent, such as it is for swimmers who participate in morning and evening practices and for soccer players who compete in tournaments. In these situations and others like them, faster glycogen replenishment translates into significantly better performance in the subsequent exercise session. This was shown in a study in which investigators tested a carbohydrate/protein drink that had a 4:1 ratio of carbohydrate to protein. The researchers found that when athletes consumed the carbohydrate/protein drink immediately after exercise, they had 55 percent greater endurance in an exercise bout four hours later when compared with the consumption of carbohydrate supplement. (See Figure 5.1.)

Confirmation of these results was obtained in a trial involving runners. One group received a carbohydrate drink, and the second received a carbohydrate/protein drink. The carbohydrate/protein drink improved run time to exhaustion by 29 percent.

The implications of this difference are pretty obvious to any aerobic athlete, from the basketball player who often plays back-to-back games on a Friday and Saturday night to the triathlete who routinely trains twice a day. By replenishing muscle glycogen stores rapidly, you have more energy the next time you work out or compete.

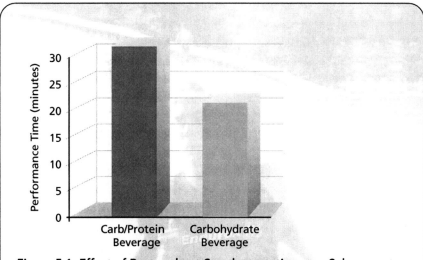

Figure 5.1. Effect of Postworkout Supplementation on a Subsequent Exercise Bout
Following a glycogen-depleting exercise bout, subjects were given either a carbohydrate or a carbohydrate/protein/antioxidant beverage. Following a four-hour recovery period, the subjects completed an exercise bout to exhaustion. When the subjects received the carbohydrate/protein/antioxidant drink, their performance times in the second workout were 55 percent better than when they received the carbohydrate supplement. *(Adapted from Williams et al.)*

Initiate Tissue Repair and Set the Stage for Muscle Growth

Protein consumption in its own right will stimulate protein synthesis by raising blood amino acid levels. Insulin, however, is also a strong stimulator of protein synthesis. When protein is taken in conjunction with carbohydrate, it stimulates protein synthesis two ways: first, by raising the blood amino acid levels, and second, by stimulating the release of insulin.

This is evidenced in a study showing a carbohydrate/protein combination was 38 percent more effective in stimulating protein synthesis than a protein supplement and more than twice as effective as a carbohydrate supplement. (See Figure 5.2.)

Another benefit of adding protein to a carbohydrate mixture is that it helps maintain glutamine levels. Glutamine, the most prevalent amino acid within muscle, plays an important role in providing energy for immune system function. During exercise, glutamine levels are severely depleted. Protein consumed postexercise maintains glutamine levels better than a carbohydrate drink.

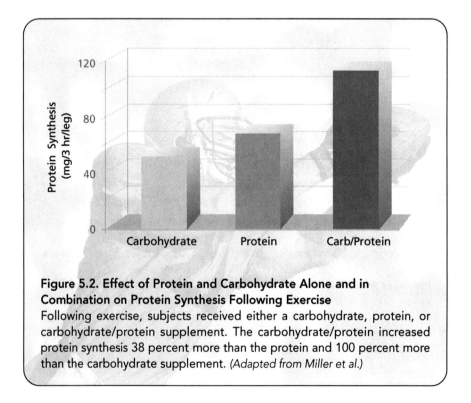

Figure 5.2. Effect of Protein and Carbohydrate Alone and in Combination on Protein Synthesis Following Exercise
Following exercise, subjects received either a carbohydrate, protein, or carbohydrate/protein supplement. The carbohydrate/protein increased protein synthesis 38 percent more than the protein and 100 percent more than the carbohydrate supplement. (Adapted from Miller et al.)

Reduce Muscle Damage and Support the Immune System

You cannot eliminate muscle damage that occurs as a consequence of strenuous exercise. You can minimize it, however, with the consumption of the right nutrients. Consuming the right nutrients postexercise can go a long way toward minimizing the extent of muscle damage. In a study, researchers from the University of North Texas showed that a carbohydrate/protein supplement significantly reduced free-radical formation, a cause of muscle damage. In a second study from St. Cloud's University, researchers found consumption of a carbohydrate/protein drink reduced blood levels of CPK (an indicator of muscle membrane damage) at twenty-four-hours postexercise by 36 percent when compared with a carbohydrate-only drink. (See Figure 5.3.)

Since strenuous exercise can compromise the immune system, researchers hypothesized that nutrient intervention postexercise may minimize this effect. Researchers at Vanderbilt University and the United States Marine Corps recently showed that following strenuous exer-

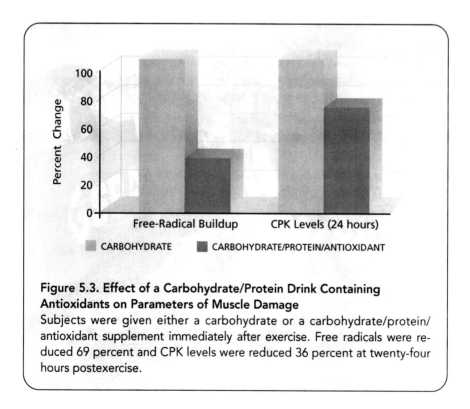

Figure 5.3. Effect of a Carbohydrate/Protein Drink Containing Antioxidants on Parameters of Muscle Damage
Subjects were given either a carbohydrate or a carbohydrate/protein/ antioxidant supplement immediately after exercise. Free radicals were reduced 69 percent and CPK levels were reduced 36 percent at twenty-four hours postexercise.

cise, consumption of a carbohydrate/protein drink reduced bacterial infections by 28 percent, reduced muscle joint problems by 37 percent, and decreased total medical visits by 33 percent when compared with a carbohydrate-only drink. These results indicate that athletes who pay attention to postexercise recovery nutrition may also be more resistant to colds because they will have a healthier immune system. The subjects who took carbohydrate/protein supplements in the Vanderbilt study also had 83 percent fewer medical visits due to heat exhaustion after strenuous exercise in hot conditions.

There have been a number of recent articles discussing why protein should *not* be in a sports drink. One of the reasons generally given is that protein tends to impede fluid replenishment. The study at Vanderbilt University actually presents a strong case that a carbohydrate/protein supplement may be *more* effective than a carbohydrate-only supplement in preventing dehydration. Although the exact cause is not known, the researchers speculated that an increase in blood amino acid levels might help speed the absorption of fluids.

Start the Replenishment of Fluid and Electrolytes

As seen in the previous chapter, because of limitations in the absorption of water, athletes may complete their exercise dehydrated even when they drink regularly throughout exercise. One of the easiest ways to determine the amount of dehydration you experience during exercise is to weigh yourself before and after exercise and calculate the difference. To ensure complete rehydration before the next day's workout, drink 1.5 ounces of fluid for every ounce of body weight you lost during exercise over the next eight to twelve hours. You should weigh yourself again before the next workout and make sure that you are within one pound of yesterday's starting weight.

Dehydration can be cumulative. In other words, the degree of dehydration worsens if fluids are not fully replenished after every workout. This is a more common problem than athletes realize. Preventing cumulative dehydration becomes extremely important in situations such as soccer tournaments in which multiple games are played in the same day and in any sport in which multiple competitions take place on consecutive days. Because of the relationship between dehydration and exercise performance, an athlete who starts a competition or workout slightly dehydrated will fatigue that much sooner.

Can Recovery Nutrition Keep You Free from Colds?

There is a clear relationship between exercise and the status of the immune system. However, it is not a simple relationship. On one hand, a number of major epidemiological studies (that is, studies involving an entire population) have shown that people who engage in mild to moderate exercise are healthier than those who do not exercise at all. Surveys of endurance athletes show that between 60 and 90 percent feel they are healthier than the average person. Epidemiological studies verify this perception. Regular exercise can reduce cold symptoms by up to 50 percent. The reason may relate to the fact that the bodies of regular exercisers adapt to the stress of exercise. The key here may be the hormone cortisol. Cortisol has been shown to have a suppressive effect on the immune system. The greater the stress on the body, the greater the cortisol release. Individuals who exercise regularly have a smaller increase in cortisol during exercise.

For people who exercise strenuously on a regular basis, the situation is far different. Studies of elite runners have shown that overtraining significantly lowers resistance to upper respiratory infections. Similar results have been shown in other sports. After hard exercise, there is a temporary compromise of immune function. During this time, an overtrained athlete may be far more susceptible to infection.

Nutrition, both during and after exercise, may prevent this temporary compromise of immune function. Carbohydrate ingestion during exercise has been shown to not only lower blood cortisol levels but also to help prevent a decrease in immune function.

A carbohydrate/protein drink may even be more effective. Researchers from Vanderbilt University and the United States Marine Corps reported that subjects who consumed a carbohydrate/protein supplement post-exercise had 28 percent fewer visits to the doctor due to bacterial or viral infections than subjects who consumed a carbohydrate supplement.

The carbohydrate/protein supplement may not only lessen the impact of cortisol and its effects, but may also help athletes maintain glutamine levels. Glutamine, the most prevalent amino acid in muscles, plays an important role in providing energy for immune system function. Strenuous exercise depletes glutamine levels, but researchers have shown that a carbohydrate/protein drink actually maintains glutamine levels.

If this chapter doesn't give you reason enough to pay attention to post-exercise nutrition to improve performance, you now have one more reason—it can keep you healthier.

GUIDELINES FOR RECOVERY NUTRITION

Nutrition has its biggest impact during the first forty-five minutes post-exercise, the metabolic window. To take advantage of this window is to optimize exercise recovery and training adaptation. Below are general guidelines for your immediate recovery nutrition. These guidelines are based on a strenuous workout that results in substantial glycogen depletion. In Chapter 6, you'll learn how to develop your personal nutrition action plan according to your activity level and training program. The ideal recovery drink to consume postexercise should composed of the ingredients listed in Table 5.1. Each of these ingredients is discussed below.

5.1. IDEAL NUTRIENT COMPOSITION FOR A POSTEXERCISE SUPPLEMENT

Nutrient Objectives	Ideal Composition (per 12 oz water)
• Shift the metabolic machinery into an anabolic (muscle-building) state from a catabolic (muscle-depleting) state	High-glycemic carbohydrates, such as glucose, sucrose, and maltodextrin: 50–60 g
	Whey protein: 14 g
• Replenish muscle glycogen stores	Glutamine: 1–2 g
• Initiate tissue repair and set the stage for muscle growth	Vitamin C: 60–120 mg
	Vitamin E: 80–200 IU
• Reduce muscle damage and support the immune system	Sodium: 100–200 mg
	Potassium: 60–100 mg
• Start the replenishment of fluid and electrolytes	Magnesium: 60–120 mg

Carbohydrate

Consume an amount of carbohydrate that will maximize muscle glycogen replenishment. High-glycemic carbohydrates are preferable to lower-glycemic carbohydrates. High-glycemic carbohydrates are rapidly absorbed and produce a strong insulin response. These types of carbohydrate are the catalysts that drive greater anabolic activity postexercise. A complex carbohydrate (that is, a low-glycemic carbohydrate), although it may be more beneficial during other parts of the day, simply will not do the job in the Performance Zone. Any combination of high-glycemic carbohydrates is effective. You should, however, avoid products that contain a large percentage of low-glycemic carbohydrates such as fructose or galactose, which are weaker stimulators of insulin.

Protein

Consume a quality protein with the carbohydrate. This will supply the needed amino acids for protein synthesis and heighten the insulin response. Insulin will stimulate muscle glycogen storage, amino acid transport, and protein synthesis while also reducing protein breakdown.

The ideal protein supplement is whey. Whey is a rapidly absorbed, high-quality protein that contains most of the essential amino acids. It is high in branched chain amino acids, which are often depleted during prolonged exercise, and it contains high levels of glutamine. Whey is inexpensive and, for the most part, is extremely well tolerated. Although whey normally contains lactose (milk sugar), to which some people are intolerant, lactose-free whey products (that is, products that contain less than a tenth of a percent of lactose) are available.

Ideal Ratio of Carbohydrate to Protein

The introduction of carbohydrate/protein recovery drinks into the world of sports has raised the question of what is the ideal ratio of carbohydrate to protein. For aerobic exercise, since replenishment of muscle glycogen is still the primary objective, the level of carbohydrate should be high enough to drive this process. A 4:1 ratio of carbohydrate to protein not only drives muscle glycogen replenishment but also stimulates other anabolic processes such as protein synthesis and muscle tissue repair.

Amino Acids

The protein in your recovery drink will give you just about all of the amino acids you need. The amino acid glutamine might be one exception. Studies have shown that there is a depletion of glutamine in working muscles, and that supplementation with glutamine may reduce the immunosuppressive effects of strenuous exercise. Consuming a carbohydrate/protein drink during exercise will certainly help maintain glutamine levels, but because of the role glutamine plays in supporting immune function, additional glutamine may offer a benefit in a recovery drink.

Antioxidants

Given the association between free-radical formation and muscle damage, antioxidants—particularly vitamins C and E—should be part of postexercise recovery nutrition.

Fluids

Replace 150 percent of the fluid lost within eight hours of exercise. Start this process as soon after exercise as possible using a supplement that contains the appropriate concentrations of electrolytes.

Table 5.2 compares the benefits of the four most commonly used beverages postexercise: water, carbohydrate/electrolyte sports drinks,

5.2. COMPARISON OF BEVERAGES USED POSTEXERCISE

Functional Activity	Water	Carbohydrate/ Electrolyte	Protein	Carbohydrate/ Protein/ Electrolyte/ Antioxidant
Restore fluids	√	√	√	√
Restore electrolytes	·	√		√
Replenish glycogen		√		√√
Stimulate protein synthesis	√		√√	√√√
Increase amino acid transport			√	√√
Prevent protein degradation		√		√√
Blunt cortisol		√		√
Maintain glutamine levels			√	√√
Stimulate insulin	√√	√		√√√
Support immune function		√	√	√√
Reduce muscle damage		√	√	√√

protein supplements, and carbohydrate/protein/electrolyte/antioxidant recovery drinks. The first column lists the physiological and metabolic activities that are necessary for a rapid and complete recovery to occur. As you can see, only when the proper combination of nutrients is included in the recovery drink is recovery optimized.

Solid Food versus Beverages

There are a number of advantages to consuming postexercise nutrition in a liquid form. Beverages are more convenient, easier to consume when you are not hungry, take care of hydration and nutrient requirements simultaneously, and can be designed to provide precisely the right combinations of ingredients.

SUMMARY

Postexercise supplementation should begin within fifteen minutes after you complete exercise or you will risk missing the metabolic window of opportunity. The key to optimum recovery is to stimulate insulin, which controls most of the muscle cells' postexercise anabolic processes. Consuming the right combination of nutrients can accelerate muscle recovery, stimulate the rebuilding of muscle protein, and reduce muscle inflammation and soreness. A combination of carbohydrate and protein is superior in helping muscles recover than either a carbohydrate or protein supplement alone.

6.
Your Nutrition Action Plan

I n the preceding chapters, we described some of the latest studies demonstrating how nutrition can improve performance and help you recover rapidly and more completely after training and competition. In this chapter, you'll learn how to create your own nutrition action plan. It's not complicated, but you'll probably have to make some changes in your approach to nutrition.

ABOUT YOUR NUTRITION ACTION PLAN

Your nutrition action plan is divided into two segments: nutrient and fluid needs before and during exercise, and nutrient and fluid needs after exercise. Keep in mind the 30W15 rule. Start nutrient intervention **30** minutes before exercise and continuing through your **W**orkout and consuming your recovery nutrition within **15** minutes after your workout. Following this rule will allow you to time your nutrition to optimize muscle performance and recovery. Keep the following important points in mind while designing your personal plan.

➤ **Never try a new nutrition practice for the first time in competition.** If you have not been drinking much during exercise prior to reading this book, begin by drinking plain water. As you become accustomed to drinking during exercise and start to approach the recommended level of fluid consumption, switch to a carbohydrate/electrolyte sports drink or preferably a carbohydrate/protein/electrolyte sports drink.

➤ **Once you create your nutrition plan, follow it consistently.** Most athletes apply discipline to their training regimen. They design their individual workouts to improve both their endurance and skill set and they follow their training program religiously. Think of nutrition as an integral part of your training. After you create your action plan, you should implement it every time you train. This will be easy to do because your behavior will be continually reinforced by the improvement in your athletic performance.

➤ **Shoot for the intake levels of nutrients and fluid recommended in this book.**

The previous chapters outline the target goals for fluid and nutrient consumption before, during, and after exercise. These target goals represent the ideal nutritional recommendations. However, there are some critical limitations that may prevent you from fully implementing all of these recommendations. The most important is that your digestive system has an "upper limit" on the amount of fluid and carbohydrate that it can absorb. Generally, the upper limit for fluid is 34–41 ounces (1,000–1,200 milliliters) per hour and the upper limit for carbohydrate is 60–72 grams per hour. It is not uncommon for athletes to lose more than 34 ounces of fluid per hour when they exercise in hot weather. Therefore, it can be physiologically difficult, if not impossible, to completely replace fluid loss during exercise. The important point is that you should still shoot for the target levels. Replenishing fluid and carbohydrate up to the maximum level that your digestive tract can absorb or the level that is feasible under the constraints of your sport or activity will result in better performance than drinking less.

CREATING YOUR NUTRITION ACTION PLAN

Every athlete is different, and therefore each has his or her own unique nutritional requirements. In this next section, we describe in four easy steps how you can tailor these general recommendations into your own nutrition action plan. It involves a few simple calculations based on your weight and your activity level. If you participate in more than one sports activity, create separate nutrition action plans for each.

1. Compute Your Total Caloric Expenditure

Figuring out your total caloric expenditure is the most important calculation you'll make. From this figure, you can determine your fluid and carbohydrate needs. Total caloric expenditure is a function of your exercise activity, the intensity and duration of your exercise, and your weight in pounds. Table 6.1 lists the energy expenditure values for a wide range of exercise activities. To determine your total caloric expenditure, select from Table 6.1 the energy energy expenditure value based on your activity and intensity. This number is multiplied by your weight in pounds and your workout duration.

For example, if you train by running at an eight-minute per mile pace, weigh 150 pounds, and exercise for forty-five minutes, your calculated caloric expenditure would be:

Total Caloric Expenditure = .09 (cal/min/lb) x 150 lb x 45 min = 607 calories

6.1. ENERGY EXPENDITURE VALUES FOR DIFFERENT EXERCISE ACTIVITIES

Activity	Energy Expenditure Value (cal/min/lb)	Activity	Energy Expenditure Value (cal/min/lb)
Aerobic: high impact	0.07	Running: 7 min/mile	0.10
Aerobic: low impact	0.04	Running: 8 min/mile	0.09
Basketball	0.06	Running: 9 min/mile	0.09
Cycling 10 mph	0.06	Running: 11.5 min/mile	0.06
Cycling 15 mph	0.08	Skiing vigorous/racing	0.06
Cycling 17.5 mph	0.09	Soccer competitive	0.08
Cycling > 20 mph	0.12	Strength Training: Circuit	0.06
Football	0.07	Strength Training: Vigorous	0.05
Golf (carrying clubs)	0.04	Swimming back stroke	0.08
Gymnastics	0.03	Swimming breast stroke	0.07
Mountain bike	0.06	Swimming freestyle*	0.06
Running, cross-country	0.07	Swimming freestyle**	0.08
Running: 5.5 min/mile	0.13	Tennis Match	0.08
Running: 6 min/mile	0.11	Volleyball	0.02

*50 yards/min   **75 yards/min

2. Calculate Your Fluid and Carbohydrate Needs During Exercise

From your total caloric expenditure value, you can calculate your nutrient and fluid needs. As you've learned, the generation of energy produces heat. Sweating is the primary mechanism by which your body cools itself. Therefore, there is a direct relationship between the amount of sweating and total caloric expenditure. Generally, your body sweats about 4.5 ounces of water for every 100 calories you expend in exercise.

Table 6.2 lists total fluid loss from sweating for a wide range of total caloric expenditure values. For an eight-minute per mile runner, the total caloric expenditure is 607 calories. In order to sufficiently cool the body, this athlete would lose about 27 ounces of fluid through sweating.

Ideally, this amount should be totally replenished. Practically, however, this might be difficult. For example, elite marathoners, on average, consume 20 ounces of water per hour, which is significantly less than they lose by sweating. Cyclists generally have an easier time in meeting the target fluid recommendations, because they have more opportunity to drink, whereas soccer players, because of the rules of the sport, would find it exceedingly difficult. We'll discuss the special nutrition challenges associated with a variety of sports in the next chapter.

Table 6.2 is also an easy way to compute your fluid needs for exercise that takes place in temperatures that do not exceed 80°F and humidity that does not exceed 60 percent. However, the following are some important caveats that will result in greater fluid loss than the amounts outlined in Table 6.2.

- **High humidity.** When humidity exceeds 60 percent, the rate of fluid loss increases. The sweat falls off the body as water rather than being evaporated, resulting in a less efficient cooling process.

- **High temperature.** When the temperature exceeds 80°F, especially on sunny days, your body begins to pick up heat from the environment, necessitating additional sweat evaporation for cooling.

- **Equipment.** The equipment and uniforms football and hockey players wear prevent normal evaporation from occurring because they absorb the sweat, rendering it unavailable for evaporation. As a general rule, hockey and football players should consume more fluids. Fortunately, frequent stoppages in play permit greater fluid consumption.

Your carbohydrate needs can be calculated as a direct percentage of your total caloric expenditure. An excellent target is to consume sufficient carbohydrate to equal 25 percent of your total caloric expenditure. For the eight-minute per mile runner, this would translate into approximately 150 calories of carbohydrate. Since 1 gram of carbohydrate equals 4 calories, this represents 37.5 grams. After you know your total caloric expenditure, use Table 6.2 to determine your carbohydrate needs during exercise. (This table is also used in Step 3.)

6.2. DETERMINING FLUID AND NUTRIENT NEEDS DURING EXERCISE

Total Caloric Expenditure (cal)	Total Fluid Loss Thru Sweating (oz)	Target Carb Caloric Intake* (cal)	Carb (g)	Protein (g)	Sports Drink** (oz)	Water (oz)	Total Target Fluid Intake (oz)
200	9	50	12.5	3.1	7	1.9	8.9
250	11	63	15.6	3.9	9	2.4	11.4
300	14	75	18.8	4.7	11	2.9	13.9
350	16	88	21.9	5.5	12	3.4	15.4
450	20	113	28.1	7.0	16	4.4	20.4
500	23	125	31.3	7.8	18	4.8	22.8
550	25	138	34.4	8.6	19	5.3	24.3
600	27	150	37.5	9.4	21	5.8	26.8
650	29	163	40.6	10.2	23	6.3	29.3
700	32	175	43.8	10.9	25	6.8	31.8
750	34	188	46.9	11.7	26	7.3	33.3
800	36	200	50.0	12.5	28	7.8	35.8
850	38	213	53.1	13.3	30	8.2	38.2
900	41	225	56.3	14.1	32	8.7	40.7
1000	45	250	62.5	15.6	35	9.7	44.7
1200	54	300	75.0	18.8	42	11.6	53.6

*25% of Caloric Expenditure   **(6% carb/1.5% protein)

Are All Sports Drinks the Same?

Products do not have to meet specific requirements in order to be labeled a sports drink. The table below lists the different types of products marketed for use during and after exercise and sports. They are divided into four categories: 1) supplemented waters (bottled waters with minerals and/or vitamins added), 2) sports drinks, 3) energy-dense recovery drinks, and 4) non-sports drinks. Generally, water and sports drinks are the beverages of choice for use during athletic activity. A quick review of the ingredients shows that supplemented waters only address the fluid needs and sometimes the electrolyte needs resulting from exercise.

Because sports drinks contain carbohydrate in a 6 to 8 percent range, they are far more effective than supplemented water, and the addition of protein provides a number of extra benefits.

Per 12 ounces	Carb (%)	Carb (g)	Protein (g)	Calories
Supplemented Water				
Pedialyte	2.5	9	—	36
Propel	1.3	3	—	15
Ultima	2.5	9	—	35
Vitamin Water	5.0	19	—	75
Sports Drinks				
Accelerade	6.5	21	5.5	120
AllSport	8.0	27	—	105
Cytomax	5.0	15	—	72
Extran	5.0	16	—	68
Gatorade	6.0	21	—	75
Gatorade Endurance	6.0	22	—	88
Powerade	8.0	27	—	105
PowerBar	7.0	25	—	105
Sobe Sport	11.0	36	—	131
Energy Dense Recovery Drinks				
Endurox R4	15.0	52	13	270
Countdown	12.0	41	14	230
Non Sports Drinks				
Regular cola	11.0	26	—	142
Orange juice	11.0	33	3	165
Red Bull	11.0	27	—	108

Energy-dense recovery drinks are among the newer nutrition products for athletes. They are specifically designed to stimulate muscle-rebuilding processes postexercise.

The last category is made up of those products that should not be (but often are) used either during exercise or postexercise. This category includes carbonated beverages, fruit juices, and caffeine-containing beverages that have an 11 percent carbohydrate content. Carbonated sodas should not be consumed either during or after exercise. After a hard workout, athletes are almost always fluid depleted. Drinking a carbonated beverage makes you feel full faster so you drink less. Also, these products usually do not contain sufficient electrolytes to fully restore those lost through sweating. Finally, there is no advantage in using a caffeine product postexercise. For more information on caffeine, see Chapter 8.

Sodium (mg)	Potassium (mg)	Magnesium (mg)	Vitamin E (IU)	Vitamin C (mg)	Caffeine
Supplemented Water					
372	282	—	—	—	—
53	—	—	3	6	—
75	150	24	—	300	—
—	—	—	—	60	—
Sports Drinks					
190	65	75	30	60	—
82	82	—	—	6	—
75	83	—	—	60	—
92	74	—	—	—	—
165	45	—	—	—	—
300	135	4	—	—	—
82	75	—	—	—	—
240	15	16	—	6	—
154	75	15	5	—	✓*
Energy Dense Recovery Drinks					
210	120	240	400	470	—
220	121	240	200	100	—
Non Sports Drinks					
51	—	—	—	—	✓
—	675	—	—	—	—
310	—	—	—	—	✓

Also contains guarana

3. Establish Your Fueling Schedule

The next step is how best to consume your carbohydrate and fluid. You can drink water and consume a concentrated carbohydrate such as a carbohydrate gel. But some gels do not contain electrolytes and therefore will not replenish the electrolytes that you lose through sweating. Your nutrition action plan during exercise should be as easy to follow as possible. That's why we recommend using a sports drink. A quality sports drink gives you the fluid, the carbohydrate, and the electrolytes your body needs, and the newer sports drinks have added protein.

Because of the additional benefits that small amounts of protein offers in terms of endurance and a faster recovery, we recommend using a sports drink that contains this nutrient. Table 6.2 lists the necessary nutrient and fluid amounts needed based on total caloric expenditure. As shown in the table, the total caloric expenditure for the eight-minute per mile runner is 607 calories. Based on this value, 27 ounces of fluid are lost during sweating and the target carbohydrate caloric consumption is 150 calories. This translates into consuming 21 fluid ounces of a 6 percent carbohydrate/1.5 percent protein sports drink plus 5.8 ounces of water.

As you can see from Table 6.2, it is only at the higher levels of total caloric expenditure that significant amounts of water should be consumed in addition to the sports drink. In general, for exercise activities resulting in a total caloric expenditure up to 750 calories, a 6 to 8 percent carbohydrate sports drink with or without protein will be more than sufficient.

Once you have determined the needed volume, set up a drinking schedule. It is best to drink smaller amounts more frequently. Consuming 27 ounces after thirty minutes of exercise would most likely make you sick, but consuming 6–9 ounces every ten to fifteen minutes is doable.

4. Determine Your Nutrient and Fluid Needs Postexercise

There are many athletes who believe that they are better able to maintain their weight by not eating after exercise. The thinking goes, "I worked hard. I burned calories. If I don't eat, I will lose weight." There are two flaws in this thinking. First, research shows that athletes who voluntarily withhold nutrition postexercise will consume those same calories over the next twenty-four hours. In other words, you will eat more at subsequent meals and your total twenty-four-hour caloric consumption will be the same whether you ate after exercising or not. But this doesn't mean that it's a wash. To the contrary, by delaying the consumption of nutrients in the critical postexercise period, you limit the ability of your muscles to recover and adapt to training. Almost every anabolic process necessary for muscle recovery and adaptation is impeded by a two-hour delay in consuming nutrition postexercise.

The total caloric expenditure value is the basis for determining your postexercise recovery needs. Within fifteen minutes after exercise, you should consume 50 percent of your net caloric deficit (the difference between total caloric expenditure during exercise and calories consumed in the form of carbohydrate during exercise) in the form of a carbohydrate and 12.5 percent as protein. This nutrient combination will turn on the anabolic switch of the muscle machinery and strongly stimulate the replenishment of muscle glycogen storage and the repair and rebuilding of muscle protein damaged as a consequence of exercise. Use Table 6.3 on page 68 to determine your net caloric deficit.

Again, the target carbohydrate for consumption during exercise is 25 percent of your total caloric expenditure value. The eight-minute per mile runner ideally should consume 150 calories (25 percent of 600 calories) of carbohydrate during an hour run at this pace. This leaves a net caloric deficit of approximately 450 calories of carbohydrate as shown in Table 6.3.

The recovery nutrition should be 50 percent of this value or 225 calories of carbohydrate. If you consume a carbohydrate/protein recovery drink, this translates into 56 grams of carbohydrate and 14 grams of protein. The most practical way to get these nutrients is in the form of a sports drink or energy-dense recovery drink. The type of beverage that you consume will determine how many ounces you will need. Table 6.4 on page 69 shows the amount of fluid you would need to consume to get the appropriate nutrient value from four different types of sports drinks containing 5 percent, 6 percent, 7 percent, and 8 percent carbohydrate as well as from two of the new energy-dense recovery drinks (12 percent and 15 percent) specifically formulated to optimize the recovery process.

When the postexercise carbohydrate requirement does not exceed 42 grams, a sports drink will usually do the job. However, as shown in Table 6.4, when the postexercise nutrient needs are higher, it becomes increasingly difficult to satisfy them with a sports drink. If the target carbohydrate consumption is 225 calories that would require 38 ounces of a 5 percent drink, or 24 ounces of an 8 percent drink but only 13 ounces of an energy-dense recovery drink that contains 15 percent carbohydrate. Many people cannot drink the large volumes of fluid that would have to be consumed in order to get adequate carbohydrate and protein from a sports drink after exercise. The new energy-dense drinks enable you to consume your calories with significantly less fluid volume.

6.3. DETERMINING POSTEXERCISE NUTRIENT NEEDS

	Total Caloric Expenditure (cal)	Target Caloric Consumption* (cal)	Net Caloric Deficit (cal)	Target Carb Consumption† (cal)	Macronutrient Composition		Sports Drink (oz)**	Recovery Drink (oz)††
					Carb (grams)	Protein (grams)		
Sports Drink	200	50	150	75	19	5	11	
	250	63	188	94	23	6	13	
	300	75	225	113	28	7	16	
	350	88	263	131	33	8	19	
	450	113	338	169	42	11	24	
Energy Dense Recovery Drink	500	125	375	188	47	12		11
	550	138	413	206	52	13		12
	600	150	450	225	56	14		13
	650	163	488	244	61	15		14
	700	175	525	263	66	16		15
	800	200	600	300	75	19		17
	900	225	675	338	84	21		19
	1000	250	750	375	94	23		21
	1200	300	900	450	113	28		25

*During exercise (25 percent of caloric expenditure)
†50 percent of net caloric deficit
**Sports Drink—6% carbohydrate/1.5% protein (ounces)
††Recovery Drink—15% carbohydrate/3.75% protein (ounces)

6.4. VOLUMES OF CARBOHYDRATE SPORTS DRINKS REQUIRED TO MEET SELECTED POSTEXERCISE NUTRIENT NEEDS

Target Carbohydrate Caloric Consumption*	Carb (g)	Sports Drink				Recovery Drink	
		5% Carb (oz)	6% Carb (oz)	7% Carb (oz)	8% Carb (oz)	12% Carb (oz)	15% Carb (oz)
188	47	32	26	23	20	13	11
225	56	38	32	27	24	16	13
244	61	41	34	30	26	17	14
300	75	51	42	36	32	21	17

*Within 15 minutes postexercise (50% of caloric deficit)

It is important to consume your postexercise nutrition within the metabolic window. Since the key to turning on the muscle's anabolic processes is insulin, an objective of your postexercise nutrition is to elevate insulin levels rapidly. Doing so in the presence of the right combination of nutrients will activate almost all of the cell's recovery processes. Drinking a sports drink that has a lower percentage of carbohydrate over a longer period of time may not generate the insulin surge necessary to turn on the muscles' anabolic switch.

There are a number of other advantages to consuming your recovery meal as a beverage. First of all, sports or recovery drinks are convenient to use and can easily be carried in a gym bag. As mentioned earlier, many athletes are simply not hungry after a workout, but they usually don't mind drinking. If you wait until your appetite is restored after a workout, you may miss the critical metabolic window of opportunity. Beverages designed specifically for recovery are easy to digest and are absorbed faster than solid food. It may take the nutrients in solid food up to one to two hours to reach the muscles.

Fully Replenish Fluid and Carbohydrate

If you do consume an energy-dense recovery drink, it is important that you continue drinking sufficient amounts of fluid to replace about 150 percent of your estimated sweat loss before your next exercise session. This will ensure complete hydration.

Similarly, if you have significantly depleted your glycogen stores during your training session, complete replenishment of muscle glycogen will require additional carbohydrate consumption during the subsequent fifteen to twenty hours of recovery. Therefore, you should try to incorporate the recovery process into your normal meal plan. The following are general recommendations for daily carbohydrate consumption:

➤ Moderate duration (1–1.5 hours per day)/low-intensity endurance training: Consume 2.5–3.0 grams of carbohydrate per pound of body weight per day.

➤ Moderate to heavy duration (1–3 hours per day)/moderate- to high-intensity endurance training: Consume 4–5.5 grams of carbohydrate per pound of body weight per day.

➤ Extreme exercise training (4–6 hours per day): Consume 4.5–6 or more carbohydrate per pound of body weight per day.

PERFORMANCE ZONE NUTRITION

By now you realize that it is easy to implement your own nutrition action plan so that when you exercise you are truly in the Performance Zone. Simply follow the 30W15 rule. The science shows that with the right combination of nutrients you can address almost all of the critical nutrition issues surrounding exercise. It is no longer just about hydration. Table 6.5 illustrates the many benefits that will be gained by consuming the right combination of nutrients during the Performance Zone.

GENERAL NUTRITION RECOMMENDATIONS

Although *The Performance Zone* focuses on nutrient intervention before, during, and immediately after exercise, serious athletes of all ages should pay special attention to the food they consume during the rest of the day. The foundation for sports performance is a healthy diet. We recommend that aerobic athletes consume a diet with the following macronutrient breakdown:

• 55 to 60 percent carbohydrate

• 15 to 20 percent protein

• 30 percent fat

6.5. PERFORMANCE ZONE NUTRITION

Time	Nutrient Objectives	Ideal Composition (per 12 oz water)
30 Minutes Before Exercise (Food and water or sports drink)	• Fully hydrate • Raise blood glucose levels	High-glycemic carbohydrate: 20–26 g Whey protein: 5–6 g Vitamin C: 30–120 mg Vitamin E: 20–60 IU Sodium: 100–250 mg Potassium: 60–120 mg Magnesium: 60–120 mg
During Exercise (Sports drink)	• Replace fluids and electrolytes • Preserve muscle glycogen • Maintain blood glucose levels • Minimize cortisol increases • Set the stage for a faster recovery	High-glycemic carbohydrate: 20–26 g Whey protein: 5–6 g Vitamin C: 30–120 mg Vitamin E: 20–60 IU Sodium: 100–250 mg Potassium: 60–120 mg Magnesium: 60–120 mg
Within 15 Minutes After Exercise (Sports drink or recovery drink)	• Shift the metabolic machinery into a muscle-building state from a muscle-depleting state • Replenish muscle glycogen stores • Initiate tissue repair and set the stage for muscle growth • Reduce muscle damage and support the immune system • Start the replenishment of fluid and electrolytes	High-glycemic carbohydrate: 50–60 g Whey protein: 12.5–15 g Glutamine: 1–2 g Vitamin C: 60–120 mg Vitamin E: 80–200 IU Sodium: 100–200 mg Potassium: 60–100 mg Magnesium: 60–120 mg

Don't Skimp on Carbohydrate

As you've learned, the primary function of carbohydrate is to serve as a fuel source for the body. Despite what you hear in the media, restriction of carbohydrate can be counterproductive, especially for aerobic athletes. A low-carbohydrate diet may not provide you with enough energy. Moreover, because of carbohydrate's role in maintaining immune function, a low-carbohydrate diet may make you more susceptible to colds and other infections.

During exercise, you should consume high-glycemic carbohydrates, also called simple sugars. However, for the rest of the day, unrefined complex carbohydrates may offer significant advantages. Examples of simple sugars are fructose and sucrose. Examples of complex carbohydrates are whole foods such as wheat, brown rice, and other grains.

Get Quality Proteins

Protein is the most talked about nutrient in sports nutrition. Because of its critical role in both the structure and function of muscles, protein—in the form or enzymes, antibodies, hormones, neurotransmitters, and cell membrane receptors—control every biochemical reaction that occurs in the body. The average sedentary adult needs to consume 0.4–0.5 grams of protein per pound of body weight per day. Today, most nutritionists recognize that athletes require more protein than the average person. We suggest 0.6–0.7 grams per pound of body weight per day. However, any time an athlete is undergoing rigorous training, there is a clear benefit to consuming increased protein up to 1.2 grams per pound of body weight per day. Some of the best food sources of protein unfortunately are high in saturated fat. Therefore, it is best to limit the amount of protein you consume from foods such as red meat and whole milk.

Don't Forget the Fat

Fat has a bad image among many athletes and rightfully so. High consumption of saturated fat is a major risk factor for cardiovascular disease. Fat, however, has many essential functions within the cells of the body. It is also an ideal energy source for extended exercise because it contains almost twice the energy of glucose per gram. Total fat should account for 30 of the daily calories in your diet. Under-consumption of fat can also be a problem. For example, when fat intake dips below 20 percent of total calories, fatigue and a weakened immune system can result.

There are three basic types of fat: polyunsaturated, monounsaturated, and saturated. Limit your intake of saturated fats to no more than about 30 percent of your total fat intake. Saturated fat is not inherently bad, as many people believe. On the contrary, it is as useful as any other fat. However, excessive saturated fat consumption increases levels of LDL cholesterol in the blood, which in turn can lead to hypertension, stroke, heart attack, and other health problems.

SUMMARY

Creating your own nutrition action plan for the Performance Zone requires implementing four simple steps: 1) compute your total caloric expenditure, 2) calculate your fluid and carbohydrate needs during exercise, 3) establish your fueling schedule, 4) determine your nutrient and fluid needs postexercise. Although Performance Zone nutrition is critical for achieving peak athletic performance, it is also important that aerobic athletes follow a healthy diet, which includes 55 to 60 percent carbohydrate, 15 to 20 percent protein, and 30 percent fat. Combining a healthy diet with nutrient intervention before, during, and after exercise will allow you to reach your full athletic potential.

7.
Sport-Specific Nutrition Tips

The principles and practices described in the preceding chapters apply to Performance Zone nutrition in all sports and exercise activities. But each sport has its own unique set of sports nutrition challenges that calls for a customized application of these universal sports nutrition guidelines. For example, high levels of nutrient intake are not tolerated as well in runners as they are in cyclists. And there are far fewer opportunities for an athlete to drink during a soccer match than there are during a basketball game, for instance.

With these unique challenges in mind, we asked leading experts—including athletes, coaches, and scientists—in more than a dozen different sports and sport categories to provide sport-specific nutrition tips. The purpose of these tips is to show you how to apply the Performance Zone nutrition action plan described in the preceding chapters to the real training and competition situations you encounter daily.

FOR BASKETBALL PLAYERS

Key challenge: *Most basketball games are decided in the last few minutes, when fatigue is a factor. Anything players can do to increase their energy level in those crucial last minutes could turn a loss into a win.*

Basketball players tend to sweat very heavily during games—up to 2 quarts per hour. Most players don't drink enough to offset these losses. But it's not that hard to do, if players are actively encouraged by their coaches to drink at every opportunity (timeouts, substitutions, and halftime).

Carbohydrate replenishment is just as important. The working muscles and the nervous system burn carbohydrate rapidly during games. As muscle glycogen and blood glucose levels drop, players lose speed, power, coordination, and concentration. When this happens, shooting percentage drops and players get lazy on defense.

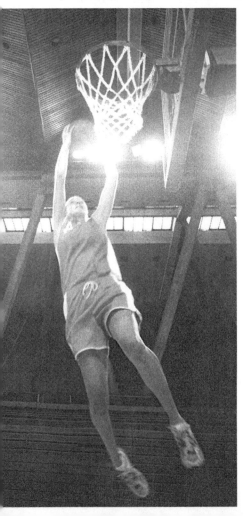

Fatigue is also a contributing factor in many of the injuries that occur on the basketball court. As players run low on energy, their form deteriorates, their reaction time slows, and they lose stability in certain joints. This leaves them much more susceptible to injury than they are when they're fresh.

A study performed at the University of Kentucky demonstrated how fatigue puts players at risk. Nineteen Kentucky women's basketball and volleyball team members took part in the study. Researchers had the players perform a series of running and rapid stopping drills. They measured the women's muscle activation patterns and ground reaction time at several points during the workout. The investigators found that muscle activation during rapid stopping was delayed when players became fatigued, rendering the knee less stable and more prone to injury.

by Rich Dalatri, C.S.C.S.

Sports drinks containing carbohydrate and protein in a 4:1 ratio have been shown to delay fatigue better than conventional sports drinks, so they're what I use with the professional players I work with. In order to maximize energy during games, I advise them to drink several ounces of a carbohydrate/protein sports drink within thirty minutes before tip-off. During the game, they should drink 7–10 ounces every fifteen minutes (real time, not game time). The exact amount they drink within this range depends on the individual player's sweat rate. (To determine your fluid needs, refer to Chapter 6.)

Halftime is generally just long enough for some muscle glycogen replenishment to occur. In order to take advantage of this opportunity, players may wish to drink 8–16 ounces of a more concentrated carbohydrate/protein recovery drink. This is an ideal formulation to use immediately after the game, too, for rapid muscle recovery.

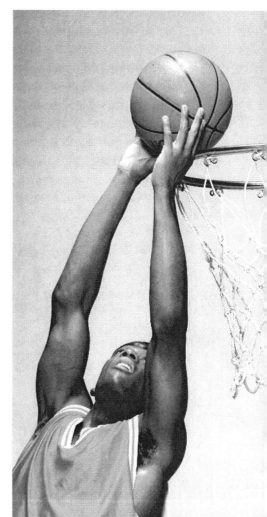

Some of the world's best basketball players now swear by the carbohydrate/protein sports drinks because they've seen that they clearly enhance their on-court performance and postgame recovery more than a traditional sports drink without protein. That second benefit is no less important given the grueling schedule of an NBA season, especially if you make the playoffs. But back-to-back games are not uncommon at all levels of play, so I urge every basketball player to use the same system I use with the game's biggest stars.

Rich Dalatri, C.S.C.S., is the strength and conditioning coach of the New Jersey Nets.

FOR CYCLISTS

Key challenge: Cycling is probably the sport in which athletes can most easily provide their bodies with the nutrition they need for maximum performance. Your squeeze bottle is within reach from start to finish. Gels and bars, if you need them, are in your rear jersey pocket. Nevertheless, even elite cyclists often make costly nutritional errors during races—witness Lance Armstrong's dehydration event during a critical time trial in the 2003 Tour de France.

The first objective of nutrition on the bike is hydration. Your hydration objective during races (and every ride, for that matter) should be to drink at approximately the same rate as you sweat. This will keep your blood volume high and maintain the efficiency of your cardiovascular system. (To determine your fluid needs, refer to Chapter 6.)

For the sake of simplicity, you can convert your drink rate into time per bottle. If you carry 24-ounce bottles and your sweat rate is 26 ounces per hour, you should drink one full bottle every fifty to sixty minutes. In hot conditions, you'll need to increase your drinking rate, of course.

Fluid empties faster from a fuller stomach, so it's helpful to drink several ounces of a sports drink a few minutes before the race begins. Then drink frequently throughout the race to keep your stomach volume and stomach-emptying rate high. For example, it's better to drink 4 ounces every ten minutes than 8 ounces every twenty minutes.

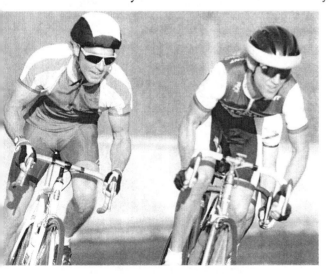

Your second nutrition objective on the bike is to take in energy. Most of this energy should come from carbohydrates. Ideally, about 20 percent of your energy intake should be in the form of proteins high in the amino acid glutamine. The addition of protein to carbohydrate provides an additional energy source, reduces muscle tissue damage, delays central fatigue, and accelerates post-ride recovery.

Cyclists should consume 250–350 calories per hour while riding. The precise amount depends on the intensity of riding and how well you tolerate nutrition intake while riding. A sports drink containing 6 percent carbohydrate and 1.5 percent protein will provide about 130 calories per 12 ounces. This concentration is just about perfect to meet your hydration and energy requirements simultaneously.

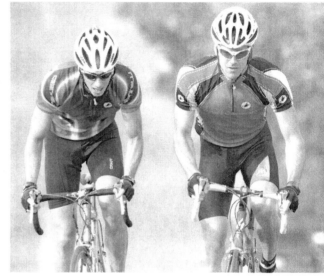

In events lasting more than three hours or so, you might want to consume something solid. Energy bars are your best choice because they travel well, contain lots of carbohydrate energy, and are easily digested. Try different brands and flavors while training in order to find out which one works best for you.

As soon as you finish a training ride or race, immediately begin to consume another 12–18 ounces of your carbohydrate/protein sports drink. This will accelerate the muscle-recovery process and allow you to resume normal training sooner.

Finally, do not neglect to drink during cold-weather rides. You may not sweat as much when it's cold, but you still sweat, and your energy needs may be even greater. By drinking the same type of sports drink at the same rate, or close to the same rate, as you do in warm weather, you will perform much better than you will without drinking. However, you will probably have to make a few more bathroom stops!

Andrew Pruitt, Ed.D., is founder and director of the Boulder Sports Medicine Institute and author of *Andy Pruitt's Medical Guide for Cyclists* (RBR Publishing Co., 2002).

FOR FOOTBALL PLAYERS

Key challenges: *There are three major nutrition challenges for football players within the Performance Zone. The first is preventing dehydration and the problems that come with it during warm-weather training and games. The second challenge is providing the muscles with the nutrition they need to delay fatigue, minimize muscle damage, and reduce the risk of injury. And the third challenge is maintaining a positive muscle protein and energy balance despite the heavy caloric demands of practices and games.*

Football players tend to be at higher risk of suffering heat illness and muscle cramps because of heavy fluid losses. Due to their large body mass, football players generate and retain more heat than smaller athletes. In addition, the helmets and heavy pads football players wear severely limit evaporative cooling.

For the sake of performance and safety, players need to make a consistent effort to hydrate throughout practices and games. Coaches need to give players free access to fluids at all times. Water is not adequate because it will not prevent the painful muscle cramps that result from

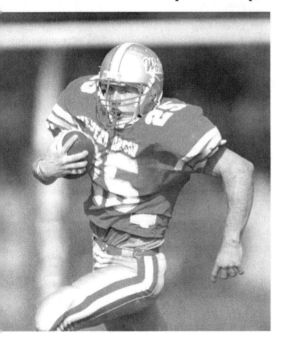

electrolyte losses. A sports drink with electrolytes will help to prevent dehydration and cramps. You can further reduce the risk of these problems by drinking consistently during the day before workouts, practices, and games.

After exercise, players should quickly rehydrate. We use weigh-ins and sweat-content information to give our players precise fluid and electrolyte benchmarks to meet postexercise. We use water, sports drinks, and electrolyte solutions such as Pedialyte to achieve rapid and complete rehydration. (To determine your fluid needs, refer to Chapter 6.)

by Jon Torine

Taking in carbohydrate within the Performance Zone is also important, but it's too little too late if you don't consume enough carbs generally. I have a system that I use with my players to ensure that their muscles are fully loaded with glycogen come game day. It starts with individually customized diet plans that are usually 55 to 60 percent carbohydrate. I also teach players to eat frequent meals and to religiously consume a carbohydrate/protein supplement after every workout and practice. In addition, I have them gradually increase their carbohydrate intake as game day approaches, in order to top off their glycogen stores.

The final step is the pre-exercise meal. Ideally, this should be a full meal (about 30 percent of the day's calories) consumed about four hours before exercise. The meal should be made up of 70 percent carbohydrates and should have an overall low-glycemic value. Although low-glycemic carbohydrates are preferable, not all of the individual carbohydrate sources have to be low-glycemic. If you have a sweet tooth (like our All-Pro receiver Marvin Harrison), you just need to be sure to take in your carbohydrates with enough protein and/or fat to slow absorption and prevent a blood-sugar crash. Some players respond well to a final carbohydrate jolt (an energy bar or carbohydrate gel) right before exercise, but this is not always necessary.

The preferred source of carbohydrate during practices and games is, of course, a sports drink, which players should consume every fifteen minutes. At halftime, I give players a carbohydrate/protein recovery drink to increase blood glucose and amino acid levels and reduce cortisol, thereby enhancing second-half endurance and minimizing muscle tissue damage.

Along with fluid and electrolytes for rehydration, carbohydrate and protein intake is also important postexercise. Consuming carbohydrate and protein within the first forty-five minutes after exercise is critical to maintaining a positive protein balance in the muscles, which is needed to maintain or increase muscle mass. It is also important for replenishing muscle glycogen so that the muscles have the energy they need for the next practice or game. The most convenient and effective way to get the needed recovery nutrition in the locker room is to have a carbohydrate/protein recovery drink waiting there. Delaying nutrient intake until the next opportunity for a sit-down meal will generally result in a compromised recovery.

Jon Torine is the strength and conditioning coach of the Indianapolis Colts.

FOR HOCKEY PLAYERS

***Key challenge:** In a hockey game, the third period is the moment of truth. If players can delay fatigue, they will be able to play harder late in the game and will have a better chance of winning.*

The primary causes of fatigue are dehydration and depletion of muscle carbohydrate stores. Adult hockey players can easily lose 3 to 6 pounds during a game—more than enough to negatively impact their performance in the third period. Youth hockey players lose a similar percentage of their body weight and with the same effect on their level of play. Carbohydrate stores also dwindle rapidly during high-intensity exercise. The average player cannot store enough carbohydrate to last an entire game, so it's important to take in additional carbohydrate during the game.

The two major consequences of fatigue on the ice are goals allowed and injuries. If it's true that fatigue contributes to injuries, we should expect to see more injuries occur early in the season, when many players are not in great shape, and late in games, when players become exhausted. A study of injuries in the United States Hockey League found that game-related injuries were more frequent during the third period, and practice-related injuries occurred most often during the first third of the season.

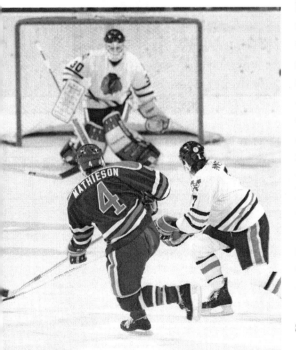

A quality sports drink can supply the fluid, electrolytes, and carbohydrate that a player needs to maintain performance in the third period. Drinking water alone will not do the job. In a study performed by researchers at the University of South Carolina, athletes who consumed a sports drink during a high-intensity hockey game were able to continue playing 45 percent longer than athletes who drank only water.

Most sports drinks are very similar. The typical sports drink contains 6 to 8 percent carbohydrate and enough electrolytes to

by John Seifert, Ph.D.

offset sweat losses. However, a new generation of sports drinks based on breakthrough research may change our idea of what constitutes the ideal sports drink. These new drinks contain a small amount of protein, which can make a big difference in performance.

The addition of protein increases the muscle's fuel efficiency by speeding carbohydrate transport into the muscle, thereby sparing muscle glycogen and delaying muscle fatigue. The result is an improvement in endurance and better maintenance of speed and reaction time. In a study my colleagues and I performed with collegiate hockey players, drinking a carbohydrate/protein drink during a ninety-minute practice improved skaters' performance by 8 percent compared with a placebo drink in a skating drill done after practice. A goalkeeper who followed the same protocol performed 11 percent better in a test of reaction time after practicing with the carbohydrate/protein drink than he did after drinking the flavored water.

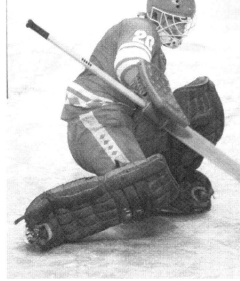

I tell the players I work with to drink about 12 ounces of a carbohydrate/protein sports drink about an hour before a game and to drink 6–10 ounces of this drink every fifteen to twenty minutes during a game. By doing this, players will be less fatigued in the third period and will be able to play harder when it really counts.

It's also important to continue drinking after the game, especially if you're playing again within thirty-six hours. The sooner you take in fluids, electrolytes, carbohydrate, and protein, the sooner your muscle will be ready for more action. Back-to-back games are common at all levels of hockey. You will perform much better in the second game if you take in the recovery nutrition you need after the first.

John Seifert, Ph.D., is associate professor of Health, Physical Education, Recreation and Sport Science at St. Cloud State University in Minnesota.

FOR LACROSSE PLAYERS

Key challenge: Lacrosse features short, high-intensity shifts, repeated sprints, full contact, and a lot of demanding upper-body work. It's truly exhausting. In addition to speed, strength, agility, and dexterity, you need to have excellent endurance to succeed as a lacrosse player. You also need to be able to recover quickly between shifts.

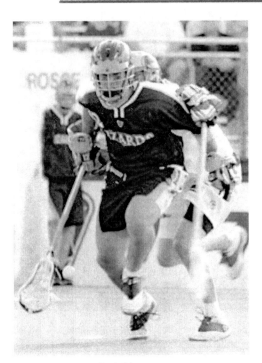

A. J. Haugen

The best way to develop the type of endurance lacrosse requires is through practice and working out. Practices should imitate the endurance requirements of game situations as closely as possible with running-based drills, frequent scrimmaging, and minimal downtime. Off-season, you need to keep in shape by running or doing other types of cardiovascular exercise several times each week.

Nutrition can be used to increase the endurance you develop in training. It starts with the pregame meal. I try to eat this meal about four hours before game time. This allows enough time for the carbohydrates I eat to make their way into my liver and muscles, but not enough time for me to get hungry again.

Between the pregame meal and the game itself, I eat nothing, but drink water regularly in order to pre-hydrate, because I sweat buckets during games, as do most lacrosse players. About twenty minutes before the game, I switch from water to a carbohydrate/protein sports drink. This tops off my blood glucose levels so that when the game begins, this becomes my muscles' main energy source, and the glycogen stored in my muscles is conserved.

by A. J. Haugen

I take a gulp our two of the same sports drink between shifts throughout the game. At halftime, I drink several ounces. I noticed a big increase in my game endurance when I switched to a carbohydrate/protein sports drink. In fact, several of my teammates are now hooked on these drinks too.

The final piece of the puzzle is drinking a carbohydrate/protein recovery drink as soon as the game is over. This has an amazing effect on muscle soreness the next day, and I recommend this practice to all lacrosse players. Sometimes we play two games in three days, or even games on consecutive days. In these situations, I feel so much better in the second game if I've taken in my recovery nutrition right after the first game. Try it!

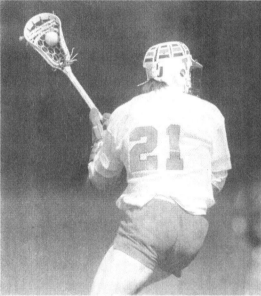

On practice days, you should follow these same basic guidelines. Eat a full meal with plenty of carbohydrates at least three hours before your practice. Hydrate as practice time gets closer, and then drink a carbohydrate/protein sports drink at regular intervals throughout the practice. Afterward, don't wait for your next sit-down meal to get the recovery nutrition you need. Have a recovery drink mixed and ready right there at the practice site. Just like your training, these nutrition practices need to be an everyday thing.

A. J. Haugen plays midfield for the Long Island Lizards of Major League Lacrosse. He is a three-time MLL All-Star.

FOR MOUNTAIN BIKERS

Key challenge: Fueling during a mountain bike race is different from fueling during a road cycling race in two important ways. First, the average intensity during a mountain bike race is usually higher. This means you sweat more and burn more fuel. Second, due to the terrain, it is harder to find opportunities to drink and easier to forget to drink.

The importance of drinking a good sports drink (and perhaps supplementing with energy gels) throughout a mountain bike race can't be overstated. In a few races, my concentration has been so focused on keeping the rubber side down and on keeping the leader in sight that I have neglected to drink as much as I should. The result has usually been premature fatigue in the critical latter stages of the race.

During many portions of a mountain bike race (for example, a rough single-track descent), it is simply not safe to take a hand off the handlebar to grab a water bottle. At other times, such as during steep climbs, it is hard to drink because you are breathing so hard. For these reasons, it is a challenge to drink on a regular schedule as you might do in a road race or running event. You just have to choose your moments carefully and make a conscious effort not to go too long without drinking.

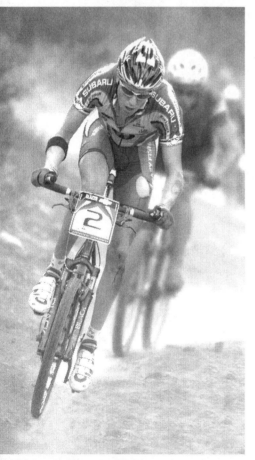

Ryder Hesjedal

Often I measure my drinking in "bottles per lap." I have a sense of how much of a full bottle I should drink between feed zones based on the length of each lap on a particular course. If I'm getting close to the feed zone and I see that my bottle is fuller than it should be, I know I need to step up my drinking rate.

by Alison Dunlap

Because there's always the possibility that you will not drink quite as much as you should during a race, it is all the more important that you start the race well hydrated and carbohydrate-loaded. I start consuming a carbohydrate/protein sports drink about ninety minutes before the start of the race and continue to drink the same mix until crossing the finish line.

If you want to return to regular training quickly after the race, it is important to make nutrition your first priority after crossing the finish line. I always have a recovery drink ready for me, and I try not to let too much time pass before I have a full meal. If I miss out on my drink and don't get a chance to eat until hours later, I feel totally flat on the bike the next day.

Of course, nutrition on the bike isn't important only during races. It's just as important during training, because the better you fuel your muscles during training rides, the better you will perform in them and the more of a fitness boost you will get from them. The only difference between my nutrition practices in races and in training rides, which are often longer, is that in the latter I tend to use more gels and energy bars. If you're out on the trails long enough, you get hungry!

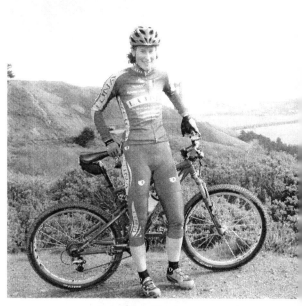

Alison Dunlap

Alison Dunlap was the 2001 cross-country mountain bike world champion and the 2002 World Cup mountain bike champion. She rides for the Luna Women's Mountain Bike Team.

FOR RUNNERS

Key challenge: In running races, it can be hard to find the right balance of nutrition intake. On the one hand, insufficient fluid and carbohydrate consumption can lead to problems such as cramping and bonking. On the other hand, too much drinking can cause other problems such as gastrointestinal discomfort.

Recently, USA Track & Field (USATF) announced a major revision in its hydration guidelines for marathon runners. In the past, USATF advised runners to drink as much fluid as possible during marathons and did not

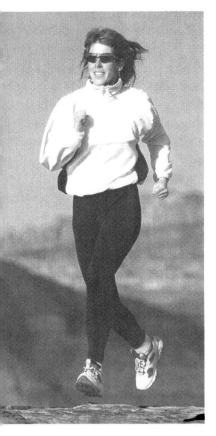

rank the hydration options of water or sports drinks in terms of preferability. The new guidelines advise runners to attempt to replace 100 percent of body fluid losses, no more, and to choose sports drinks over water.

The main impetus for the revision is the dramatic rise in cases of hyponatremia in marathons in recent years. Hyponatremia is a dangerous condition that results when the sodium concentration in the blood becomes too low. In athletes, it tends to develop in long events, when large amounts of sodium are lost through sweating and too much water is consumed, diluting the blood. Symptoms include dizziness, muscle cramping, confusion, and stomach bloating. Severe cases can lead to seizure and death. (To determine your fluid needs, refer to Chapter 6.)

When exercising at higher intensities and/or in warmer temperatures, remember that you will need to increase your rate of fluid consumption somewhat. Of course, when you drink from plastic cups handed to you by volunteers in a marathon, it's impossible to know exactly how much you're drinking. But if you have made the effort to quantify your fluid needs in training, you will be able to closely match this rate of fluid consumption by feel.

by Jeff Galloway

Note that faster and more competitive runners cannot and generally do not need to replace 100 percent of fluid losses. They should still use sports drinks instead of water, but they should drink only as much as they can get down without slowing their pace or suffering gastrointestinal discomfort. Studies show that elite marathoners drink only about 6.6 ounces (200 milliliters) of fluid per hour, although they may sweat at six or more times this rate. Sub-elite and top-tier age-group runners need to drink a little more, perhaps 10–13 ounces (300–400 milliliters).

One drawback of marathon fluid stations is that they offer only one brand of sports drink and it might not be a very good one. For example, one brand of sports drink that sponsors and is therefore served at a few major marathons contains less than 2 percent carbohydrate, which is woefully inadequate. A sports drink should contain some protein in order to further boost endurance and reduce muscle damage. But very few running events offer protein-containing sports drinks at aid stations.

In races serving such inadequate sports drinks, you might be better off carrying energy gels instead, and washing these down with water from aid stations. Carry one gel packet per half hour of racing you anticipate. Try various brands and flavors in training and choose your favorite for the race. There is now at least one brand of energy gel that contains protein.

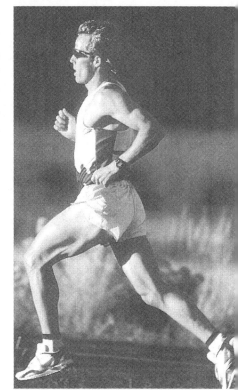

Within forty-five minutes of completing the race, be sure to drink at least 12 ounces of a sports drink or performance recovery drink containing carbohydrate and protein in a 4:1 ratio. This will result in faster muscle tissue repair and fluid and glycogen replenishment.

Jeff Galloway is the creator of the famous run-walk-run method of training and competing. He coaches thousands of runners to successful marathon finishes each year. He represented the United States at 10,000 meters in the 1972 Olympics.

FOR SOCCER PLAYERS

Key challenge: *Soccer matches are long and involve infrequent stoppages, few substitutions, and substantial amounts of high-intensity action. Therefore, soccer matches often result in large fluid losses due to sweating and significant depletion of muscle glycogen stores.*

Late in the game, players tend to become dehydrated and fatigued. This can lead to costly mistakes (goals allowed) and injuries. Approximately 30 percent of goals are scored in the last fifteen minutes of games. In the France World Cup, nearly 50 percent of all goals scored in the quarterfinals, semifinals, and final match were scored in the last twenty minutes of each game.

Recently, my colleagues and I completed a three-year study on youth soccer injuries. We found that nearly 25 percent of soccer injuries occur during the last ten to fifteen minutes of games. This is similar to findings in the Premier League in England. Fatigue appears to be an important factor in the disproportionate occurrence of injuries late in matches. When players get tired, their reaction time slows and their judgment deteriorates.

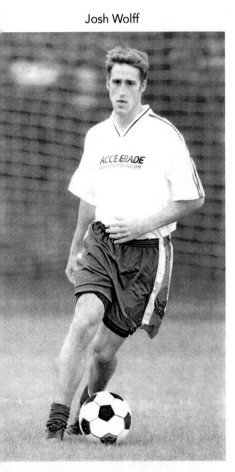

Josh Wolff

The best way to limit net fluid losses and conserve muscle glycogen stores is, of course, to frequently consume a sports drink throughout games. However, due to the infrequency and brevity of stoppages and the sheer size of the playing field, drinking opportunities can be few and far between.

In order to maximize these opportunities, teams should arrive at each game supplied with at least one large squeeze bottle per player filled with a cold sports drink. Several bottles should be placed around the perimeter of the field, a couple of bottles in each goal, and several more at the bench. Coaches should encourage

by Don Kirkendall, Ph.D.

their players to drink from the nearest bottle once every ten to fifty minutes, when an opportunity presents itself. The hotter the weather, the more frequently players should drink.

At halftime, players should drink at least 6–8 ounces of a sports drink. It is also helpful to drink several ounces within ten minutes before the start of a game. Remember, not all sports drinks are the same. A fluid and electrolyte drink is not the same as a carbohydrate replacement drink. Tests have shown that sports drinks containing carbohydrate and protein in the right balance are most effective in keeping carbohydrate levels up. (Most sports drinks have no protein.) The carbohydrate provides the fuel source while the protein helps get the fuel into the muscles more quickly.

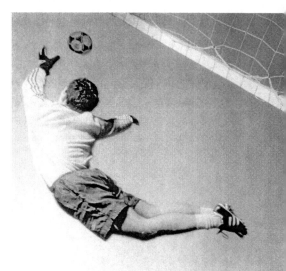

A recent study performed at St. Cloud State University compared the effects of a sports drink containing carbohydrate and protein to a sports drink containing only electrolytes on sprinting speed at the end of a long training session. Following an intense workout of seventy-five minutes, the subjects participated in four speed trials with five minutes of rest after each sprint. Half the players drank the carbohydrate/protein drink while the other half drank an electrolyte-only drink. The carbohydrate/protein group actually improved their speed by 1.1 seconds between the first and last sprints, while the other group decreased their speed by 2.2 seconds.

As soon as the game is over, players should consume another 10–16 ounces of a carbohydrate/protein sports drink to accelerate muscle recovery. This is especially important in tournament situations when another game might follow in the afternoon or next morning.

Don Kirkendall, Ph.D., is an exercise physiologist. He is a member of the U.S. Soccer Sports Medicine Committee and is on the editorial board of *Soccer Journal*.

FOR SWIMMERS

Key challenge: It is not uncommon for swimmers to race four to six times in a single meet. Swimming all-out so frequently can lead to fatigue and substandard performances in later races. Therefore, maintaining high energy levels should be a top priority for swimmers when racing more than twice in a day.

A well-conditioned swimmer has enough stored glycogen fuel to last an hour or two when doing easy lap swimming, but just one fifty-yard sprint can use up to 30 percent of a swimmer's glycogen supply.

The lower a swimmer's glycogen level drops, the more performance suffers. For this reason, swimmers must refuel their muscles with a sports drink containing plenty of carbohydrate and protein after each race. In one university study, athletes who consumed a sports drink were able to do 50 percent more sprints at maximum power than athletes who drank only water.

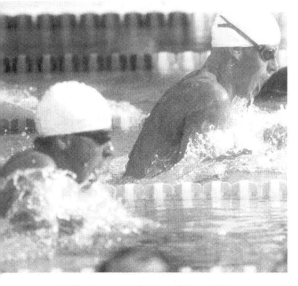

It is important to keep your muscle glycogen stores as high as possible by consuming a carbohydrate-rich diet. The most important time to take in carbohydrate is right after you finish a workout. You'll swim much better in the next workout if you're disciplined about getting the nutrition you need as soon as you finish training.

Although swim meets can last five to seven hours, it's not always possible to eat a normal meal in the middle of a meet. A full stomach diverts blood flow away from the muscles, and it can make a swimmer feel heavy and sluggish. Also, the nervousness that many swimmers experience (including me!) during meets can make eating solid foods difficult.

by Josh Davis

When there is a long break between heats or events, I like to eat a small carbohydrate-rich and easily digested food such as a banana or a whole-grain bagel. A few of these snacks in combination with regular

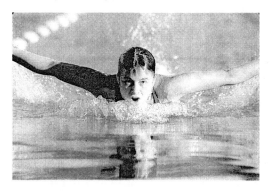

doses of a good sports drink with protein gives swimmers all the energy they need to perform at their best until the very last race is over.

Because you aren't drinking during exercise as runners and cyclists must do, you can use a more nutrient-dense performance recovery drink instead of a regular sports drink. I mix up mine in a gallon jug and carry it with me to practices and meets. The rest of the day, I sip from a gallon jug of distilled water. Some people think I'm a little fanatical about hydration and sports nutrition, but I know what a difference it makes, so I say, "Go ahead—call me weird!"

Josh Davis has won five Olympic medals and a world championships title (400m freestyle) in swimming. He has twice set the American record in the 200m freestyle.

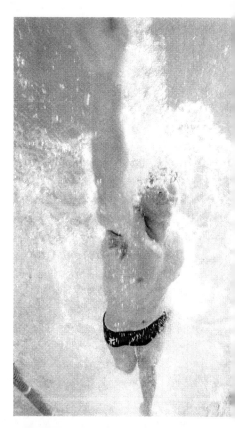

FOR TRACK AND FIELD ATHLETES

Key challenge: Track and field athletes routinely compete in multiple events and/or multiple heats during meets lasting two to four hours. These demands can leave athletes fatigued by the time the finals or their last event takes place, resulting in poor performance. Proper nutrient intervention is needed to keep athletes strong through the very last race, jump, or throw.

Most track and field athletes think of sports drinks as something distance runners need during long workouts, and that's about it. However, research shows that a single 100-meter sprint can reduce muscle glycogen by 20 percent. Sprinters competing in multiple heats and events can easily burn enough muscle glycogen—especially in their fast-twitch muscle fibers—to negatively affect performance by the end of the meet. The same is true of middle-distance and distance runners and even of jumpers and throwers.

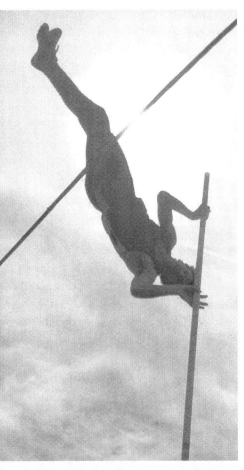

By drinking several ounces of a sports drink or recovery drink after heats, rounds, and events, track and field athletes can quickly replenish muscle glycogen and maintain glycogen levels adequate for optimal performance throughout the meet.

Sports drinks containing a proper balance of carbohydrate and protein are preferable because they have been shown to replenish glycogen faster than regular sports drinks and cause a greater improvement in performance in subsequent exercise. The amino acids in such a drink also help to maintain cell-membrane integrity and reduce muscle damage during competitive action and to repair the damage that does occur.

by Joe Vigil, Ph.D.

Staying hydrated during meets is equally important. As little as 2 percent dehydration can affect performance. Even though you might compete for only a few total minutes during a meet, that activity combined with simply being outdoors for several hours in warm air could lead to 2 percent dehydration or more without fluid intake. Keeping a bottle at hand throughout the meet and drinking according to your thirst is usually sufficient.

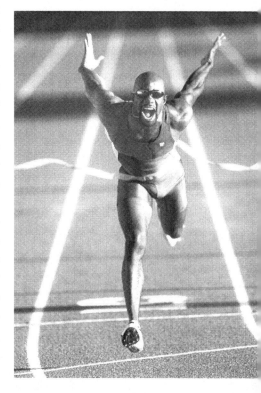

Recovery nutrition is also important. The sooner athletes can consume fluids, carbohydrate, and protein after both meets and practices, the faster and more completely they will recover from their efforts. They will have more energy, will be less sore, and will perform better in their next workout.

I've been coaching for many years and I did not always teach my athletes to practice these sports nutrition methods. When I did start to encourage my athletes to replenish fluids and carbohydrate during meets to consume timely recovery nutrition, I noticed an immediate and significant difference, and so did they.

Joe Vigil, Ph.D., is co-head coach of Team USA California. Previously, he coached at Adams State College for twenty-nine years and won nineteen NCAA Division II National Championships titles, produced 425 All-Americans, and won fourteen Coach of the Year awards.

FOR TRIATHLETES

Key challenge: A triathlon strings together three different sports that require three different fueling strategies. Therefore, the key nutritional challenge is executing the appropriate nutrition strategy in each leg of the race.

The main constraint of the swim leg is, of course, the virtual impossibility of taking in nutrition during it. For this reason, it's important that you begin the race with high levels of muscle glycogen and blood glucose. You can maximize muscle glycogen by exercising lightly or not at all on the last day or two before the race and by eating carbohydrate-rich meals the day before and the morning of the race. You can maximize your blood glucose level by drinking a few ounces of sports drink or eating a gel packet ten minutes before your wave starts.

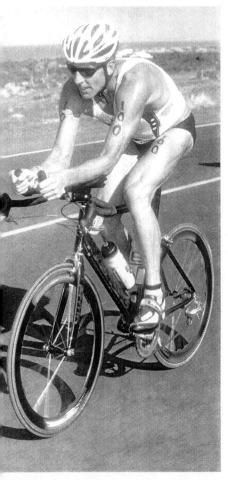

Dave Scott

On the cycling leg, it's easy to get all the nutrition your body can use. Try to consume fluids at a rate that's equivalent to at least 70 percent of your sweat rate. (To determine your fluid needs, refer to Chapter 6.)

It's also important to consume plenty of carbohydrate to supplement your body's limited glycogen stores, which are burned quickly at race intensity. The liver can only release glucose into the bloodstream at a maximum rate of about 1 gram per minute, which you can achieve by consuming 80 grams of carbohydrate per hour. If you get all of your fluid in the form of a sports drink containing 6 to 8 percent carbohydrate, you will easily achieve this rate of carbohydrate intake. However, you can get more total energy by consuming a sports drink that contains protein as well as carbohydrate.

Sports drinks are ideal and sufficient

by Siri Lindley

for your nutritional needs in sprint and middle-distance triathlons. In races lasting longer than three hours, you may want to supplement your sports drink with the use of energy bars or possibly even "real" food. This is because you might actually get hungry during long races and will want to fill some space in your rumbling gut, or because you might wish to avoid or minimize the stomach sloshing that can happen when you consume only liquids for hours on end. Most triathletes racing in a half or full Ironman use a combination of sports drink and gels or bars. A sensible ratio of liquid to solid calories is about 3:1 in long triathlons.

When running, it is impossible to drink at the same rate you can on the bike without causing gastrointestinal distress. However, your sweat rate and rate of carbohydrate burning are actually higher on the run. So the best strategy is simply to drink a sports drink at the fastest rate you can comfortably tolerate throughout the run. Drinking small amounts frequently (2–3 ounces every ten to twelve minutes) is preferable to drinking larger amounts less frequently.

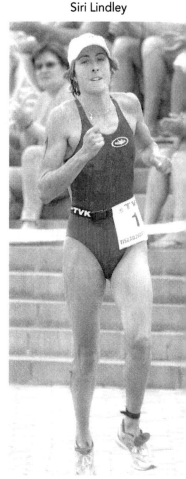

Siri Lindley

You can supplement your carbohydrate intake by swallowing a gel packet every thirty to forty minutes. Be sure to wash down the gel with water, not a sports drink, lest the carbohydrate concentration of your stomach contents become too high, resulting in slower gastric emptying and possible gastrointestinal discomfort.

For a quicker recovery after the race, drink some more of your carbohydrate/protein sports drink.

Siri Lindley is a former triathlon world champion in 2001 who was also ranked #1 in the world from 2001–2003. She now coaches triathletes in Boulder, Colorado.

FOR WINTER-SPORT ATHLETES

Key challenge: Athletes who routinely use a sports drink while practicing or competing in the summer heat are much less likely to do so while enjoying winter sports activities such as skiing, snowboarding, and skating. There is a tendency to assume that nutrition is not an important issue in cold-weather exercise. But in reality, it is just as important. Failure to use a sports drink carries the same risks in the cold as it does in the heat: dehydration, bonking, and even fatigue-related injury.

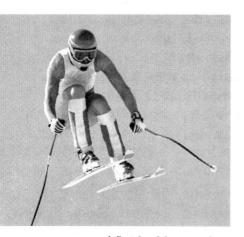

Several factors increase the likelihood of dehydration in the cold. First, cold air tends to be very dry, especially at higher altitudes, and in dry air, more fluid is lost as vapor through breathing. Second, the cold tends to suppress thirst. Even though drinking a sports drink is more palatable than water, in the cold, athletes are likely to drink less than they need. Third, cold-induced diuresis leads to a rapid fluid loss via urination, which often reduces the amount of fluid athletes voluntarily choose to drink. Finally, the heavier clothing that is worn during cold-weather activities in some winter sports not only traps heat (as it is supposed to do), but can also make movement more cumbersome and inefficient, leading to fluid loss through sweating that is comparable to that in the temperate environment.

Although winter sports are not well studied, one investigation showed that cross-country skiers experience an average of 3 percent reduction in body weight during a race—more than enough to impair performance. In another study, only two hours of slalom training resulted in a considerable weight loss when no fluids were ingested.

As in hot-weather exercise, water is not sufficient for hydration during exercise in the cold. Along with water, electrolytes (mainly sodium) are also lost in sweat. In addition, carbohydrate fuel is used for energy at high rates during winter sports activities. Thus, carbohydrate should be consumed along with fluids and electrolytes to delay fatigue that may occur through energy depletion.

by Nanna Meyer, Ph.D.

Winter-sport athletes can get the fluid and energy they need by using the same sports drinks that are used by other athletes in warm-weather and indoor sports. The difference is that the sports drink should be heated before exercise and kept warm inside a light thermos or a tightly sealed bottle wrapped in an insulating warmer. A warm sports drink is easier to drink in freezing temperatures and may help maintain core body temperature.

Alpine and freestyle skiers and snowboarders can leave their thermoses at the top or bottom of the slope and drink from them before or after runs at fifteen- to twenty-minute intervals. Cross-country skiers and snowshoers should carry their bottle (upright, if possible) in a backpack or fluid belt. Speed skaters can easily drink from bottles placed to the side of the ice. Typically, speed skaters do not need to heat their fluids if training and competition is held on indoor tracks. It is also helpful to carry convenient carbohydrate-rich snacks such as energy bars and eat them during breaks.

During long workouts on ice or long days on the slopes, sports drinks that contain small amounts of protein (such as Accelerade) may help reduce muscle protein breakdown during exercise, in addition to ensuring carbohydrate availability and maintaining fluid balance.

Ingesting fluids and foods after the workout is an integral strategy for optimizing sports nutrition in winter-sport athletes, as it helps rehydrate, speed up glycogen repletion, and stimulate protein synthesis. Skiers, snowboarders, and speed skaters should drink 17–25 ounces (500–750 milliliters) of a sports drink with electrolytes that provides 1 gram of carbohydrate per kilogram of body weight (1 kg = 2.2 lbs). The addition of small amounts of protein in liquid or solid form can further assist in the recovery process. Fluid needs for rehydration of cross-country skiers may be somewhat higher. Assessing body weight before and after the training session can best individualize fluid replacement strategies. Typically, 150 to 200 percent of lost fluids should be replaced after exercise. (To determine your fluid needs, refer to Chapter 6.)

Nanna Meyer, Ph.D., is a sports dietitian and exercise physiologist at the Orthopedic Specialty Hospital, Institute for Sport Science and Medicine, in Salt Lake City, Utah. She currently consults with U.S. Speed Skating and is a former member of the Swiss National Ski Team.

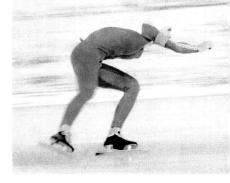

Nutrition Focus

IMPROVING BODY COMPOSITION

Most athletes in most sports benefit from having a lean body composition (that is, a low body-fat percentage). This is because muscle is the only tissue capable of performing work in any sport, whereas body fat is just dead weight. Any extra body fat beyond the amount that is required for good health reduces the efficiency of movement.

Despite their disparate appearances, 120-pound elite runners such as Kenenisa Bekele and 255-pound professional football players like Jevon Kearse have more or less the same body composition (about 5 percent body fat). The same patterns hold for female athletes in various sports. Of course, few elite athletes spend much time worrying about their body composition. For them, achieving the ideal body composition is simply a byproduct of world-class training and proper diet acting on one-in-a-million genetics.

Many other athletes, however, have a less-than-ideal body composition and would benefit from trying to improve it. How is this done?

The first step is to establish a starting point and a target. Having your body composition tested allows you to pursue the goal of improving it objectively. Two testing methods are relatively inexpensive and convenient. One option is to have an exercise physiologist or personal trainer estimate your body-fat percentage using a plastic caliper to take skin-fold measurements.

A second option is to purchase a body-fat tester for home use. These devices use bioelectrical impedance to estimate body composition with reasonable accuracy. Expect to pay about $60 for one of these devices, which you can use as often as you like.

The American Council on Exercise offers the following guidelines for body-fat percentage in men and women:

BODY-FAT PERCENTAGE GUIDELINES

	Men	Women
Athletic Range	6 to 13 percent	14 to 20 percent
Fitness Range	14 to 17 percent	21 to 24 percent
Acceptable Range	18 to 25 percent	25 to 31 percent

Once you determine your own body-fat percentage, set incremental goals to make your way to the desired range, if necessary. For example, if you're above the acceptable range, don't shoot for the athletic range right away. Aim to reach the lower end of the acceptable range. Then, once you're in the acceptable range or if you're already there, aim for the fitness range, and so on.

The optimal body-fat percentage differs among individuals. Not every athlete is genetically capable of reaching the lower end of the athletic range, and no athlete should try too hard to get there. Body-fat percentages below the athletic range are unhealthy. A level of 2 to 4 percent body fat in men and 10 to 12 percent in women is essential for normal functioning.

There are two ways to improve body composition. One way is to lose body fat and the other is to gain lean muscle mass. For example, if you weigh 200 pounds and you're carrying 30 pounds of body fat, your body-fat percentage is 15 (that is, $30 \div 200 \times 100 = 15$ percent). If you were to lose 5 pounds of body fat, your body-fat percentage would drop to 12.8 (that is, $25 \div 195 \times 100 = 12.8$ percent). If you were to gain 5 pounds of muscle and did not gain any fat, your body-fat percentage would decline to 14.6 (that is, $30 \div 205 \times 100 = 14.6$ percent). Which of these two changes is more important for you depends in part on your sport. Endurance athletes need powerful muscles but they also need to keep their total body weight low, so for them, reducing body fat is usually the priority. Strength-oriented athletes such as football and rugby players, power hitters in baseball, and throwers in track and field need a lot of raw strength, so increasing lean muscle mass is usually the priority for them. But many athletes can benefit from losing body fat and gaining lean muscle mass simultaneously.

INCREASING LEAN MUSCLE MASS

In order to gain lean muscle mass, there are three things you need to do:

1. Strength train.

2. Maintain a slight positive caloric balance.

3. Increase protein intake.

It is not enough to do just one or two of these things. Only the combination of all three is sufficient to stimulate significant muscle gains. Obviously, if you are not currently engaged in a consistent resistance-training program, you should start one. If you are already engaged in one, you may need to increase the frequency, intensity, and/or modify the format of workouts.

In order to add new tissue to your muscles, you need to maintain a positive caloric balance (that is, consume more calories than you expend) on a daily basis. However, this positive caloric balance should be slight—only 100–200 calories per day. Muscle growth is a slow process, and overeating won't make it any faster. Any extra calories you consume beyond what can be used to build new muscle tissue will probably be stored as fat.

Muscle tissue is composed mainly of protein, so protein intake needs to be prioritized. Research has shown that consuming 0.9–1.2 grams of protein per pound of body weight on a daily basis is ideal for building muscle. Overall, protein should account for 19 to 26 percent of your daily calories.

LOSING BODY FAT

A gain in lean muscle mass often results in a decrease of body fat, because it raises the resting metabolic rate (the rate at which your body burns calories at rest). As you gain muscle, your fat stores are burned to fuel the extra muscle. In addition to building muscle, there are two other things you can do to lose body fat:

1. Increase aerobic exercise.
2. Maintain a slight negative caloric balance.

As an athlete, you are already getting regular aerobic exercise, but you might benefit from doing more. For example, if you are a soccer player whose team has two practices and one game each week, you might start to do aerobic workouts (for example, jogging or cycling) on a couple of your off days at least. This additional training will not only make you a leaner athlete but will also greatly increase your endurance on the field.

Just as athletes who are trying to gain muscle need to consume 100–200 more calories than they burn each day, athletes who are seeking to lose fat need to consume 100–200 fewer calories than they burn. It is possible to achieve this slight caloric deficit simply by increasing your aerobic exercise. If not, just a few small dietary modifications will do the trick. These can include replacing sodas and fruit juices with water, substituting skim-milk dairy products for whole-milk dairy products, and replacing high-calorie snacks such as potato chips with low-calorie snacks such as fruit.

Do not cut back on nutritional supplementation within the Performance Zone. This will not help you lose fat. If anything, it will do the opposite. By fueling your exercise properly, you will be able to perform at higher levels for longer periods and burn more calories. By fueling your recovery properly, you will put calories to their best anabolic use. Studies have shown that proper supplementation during the forty-five-minute postexercise window decreases body fat in the long term, whereas consuming the same number of calories in the day without supplementation during the forty-five-minute window leads to an increase in body fat.

No matter what your sport is, it pays to be lean. The right genes can make it relatively easy to maintain an ideal body composition. But any athlete can achieve his or her individual optimum body composition with the right training and dietary regimens.

8.
Nutritional Supplements and Drugs

U se of nutritional supplements and even drugs by athletes in all sports to improve performance has become depressingly commonplace. A look at trends among younger athletes indicates this practice may become even more widespread in the coming years.

According to recent surveys, use of nutritional supplements and performance-enhancing drugs among college and high school athletes is on the rise. Results from the latest National Collegiate Athletic Association (NCAA) survey indicate that 42 percent of student-athletes use one or more types of supplement, and of these, 62 percent began supplementing in high school. A survey of male high school athletes in Louisiana showed that nearly 50 percent had tried a supplement at least once.

What is troubling about this situation is that many athletes are using supplements and drugs without adequate knowledge of their true effects—and possible side effects. And in many cases, athletes are using supplements and drugs that are banned by sport governing bodies or are both banned and illegal. It is clear that athletes are by and large poorly educated concerning the true effects of the nutritional supplements and drugs they use and their status with respect to the rules of their sport. Not all supplements are illegal or dangerous, but proper education should precede the choice to use even those supplements that are benign and condoned by the International Olympic Committee (IOC), the NCAA, and scholastic athletic associations.

This chapter reviews the effects, risks, and legal status of a variety of products that are sold to improve athletic performance. These products have been divided into two categories, those that appear safe and for which the available research substantiates a benefit, and those that should be avoided because they are ineffective and/or unsafe and/or banned by major sports organizations.

NUTRITIONAL SUPPLEMENTS THAT ARE GENERALLY SAFE AND MAY OFFER BENEFITS

All of the following substances are generally safe when used properly. Some also have proven performance benefits for some types of athletes in certain circumstances. Others require further study.

Branched Chain Amino Acids (BCAAs)

The three branched chain amino acids, leucine, isoleucine, and valine, are essential amino acids, which means they cannot be synthesized by the body and must therefore be consumed in food. These amino acids not only serve as precursors for the synthesis of other amino acids but also can be used as a direct source of energy during exercise and play an essential role in the synthesis of muscle protein following exercise.

BCAAs are abundant in many protein sources, especially whey protein. Consuming proteins that are high in BCAAs may offer a number of advantages in helping delay fatigue. The primary cause of fatigue in endurance events is depletion of muscle glycogen stores. By stimulating insulin, protein helps preserve muscle glycogen stores. In addition, the BCAAs within protein may affect other factors that play a role in the development of central nervous system fatigue (also known as central fatigue), which can affect athletes during particularly long workouts and competitions.

The best way to consume BCAAs during exercise is in a sports drink containing whey protein, which is composed of 17 percent BCAAs.

Caffeine

Caffeine is a naturally occurring chemical compound that functions in the body mainly as a mild nervous system stimulant. For decades, athletes of all kinds have used caffeine—sometimes referred to as the world's most popular drug—to enhance performance. The popularity of caffeine as a performance aid started to rise more than twenty-five years ago when Dr. David Costill of Ball State University reported that caffeine could improve endurance performance. The improvement was thought to be due to caffeine's ability to increase fat oxidation and spare the use of muscle glycogen. While this is still a possible explanation, recent research suggests that caffeine may also delay fatigue by reducing an athlete's perception of effort. Research has found that caffeine increases the concentration of hormone-like substances in the brain called ß-endorphins during exercise. The endorphins affect mood, reduce perception of pain, and create a sense of well-being.

Caffeine supplementation has also been popular among sprint and strength athletes. Although the effect of caffeine on speed and strength performance has been less tested than the effect of caffeine on endurance, the majority of research that has been done has clearly shown that there is no benefit.

Regular users of caffeine often develop a tolerance over time that will minimize any potential impact on performance it might otherwise provide. In addition, there is a wide range of individual responses to caffeine: some athletes are "low responders" and others are "high responders." The other issue is testing. The NCAA imposes a maximum limit of 15 micrograms per milliliter of caffeine in the urine, so it's best for collegiate athletes not to tempt fate and to avoid using caffeine before competitions.

There is a strong agreement among nutritionists that caffeine intake by children should be strictly limited, and this includes the use of caffeine as a performance aid by child athletes. Many kids consume "energy drinks" such as Red Bull that contain caffeine. These beverages are not sports drinks and should not be used as such for reasons beyond just their caffeine content (carbonation, high fructose content, low electrolyte content, likeliness to cause gastrointestinal discomfort, and so on).

Creatine

Creatine phosphate (CP) is an indirect source of energy that is present in muscle cells. CP can be broken down very quickly and efficiently—much more so than carbohydrate or fat—and is therefore the muscles' preferred ATP replenishment source for maximum-intensity and near-maximum-intensity efforts. However, CP is available in very limited amounts.

CP can be manufactured from its constituent amino acids in the liver and through dietary consumption of creatine, which is found in animal foods such as beef. But creatine supplementation can significantly increase the amount of CP that is stored in the muscles.

In the early 1990s, creatine exploded in popularity among athletes in strength and speed sports, bodybuilders, and recreational strength trainers when research demonstrated that creatine supplementation could increase the strength and muscle mass gains associated with consistent strength training. Creatine (usually taken in the form of creatine monohydrate) is now the most popular muscle-building nutritional supplement.

Many studies have demonstrated that creatine supplementation will enhance training-induced gains in muscle strength and mass. For example, subjects placed on creatine throughout a ten-week strength-training program increased maximal strength by 20 to 25 percent and muscle mass by 60 percent more than subjects placed on a placebo. It was also reported that college football players who supplemented with creatine and glucose during twenty-eight days of conditioning had greater gains in body weight, muscle mass, and strength compared with players who received a placebo.

There is little evidence that creatine supplementation enhances the performance of athletes in sports other than strength sports like football. Some studies have shown that creatine supplementation can improve performance in multiple-sprint workouts. Most studies involving endurance athletes have shown either no effect on performance or a negative effect, probably due to the weight gain that is typically associated with creatine supplementation.

Glucosamine and Chondroitin

Glucosamine and chondroitin sulfate are natural compounds that the body uses as building blocks for the formation of a variety of soft tissue structural elements, including the cartilage that is found in joints. Joint cartilage covers the ends of the bones that form the joint and serves to minimize friction and absorb shock during movement. Over the long term, various form of exercise can damage and wear away the cartilage in joints such as the shoulder and knee, potentially resulting in osteoarthritis.

Some research has shown that supplementation with glucosamine and chondroitin sulfate can prevent cartilage breakdown. One such study investigated the effects of glucosamine sulfate supplementation over a three-year period. This double-blind placebo-controlled study tested the effectiveness of a daily dose of 1,500 milligrams of glucosamine sulfate compared to a placebo. The results indicated a reduction in pain, increased mobility, and reduced cartilage damage.

Fewer studies have investigated the effect of supplementation with chondroitin sulfate. In one study, subjects with osteoarthritis of the knee received either 400 milligrams of chondroitin sulfate twice daily or a placebo for six months. Again, the group that received the supplementation achieved a reduction in pain and an increase in mobility.

However, none of the research conducted thus far is considered definitive. The National Institutes of Health is currently undertaking the largest and most comprehensive study of the effects of supplementation with these two compounds, but the results are not yet available.

Many distance runners, aware of the potential damage to knee cartilage, take a glucosamine or combined glucosamine/chondroitin sulfate supplement daily. To date, no study has investigated the prophylactic use of such supplements by athletes, but a majority of experts now believe that such research, when it is done, will reveal a moderate benefit.

One drawback to glucosamine supplementation is that taking this substance in high concentrations can result in insulin resistance. Athletes should be aware of this because insulin resistance can slow muscle recovery, particularly the replenishment of muscle glycogen stores.

Glutamine

As you've learned, glutamine is the most abundant amino acid in muscle cells and has been shown to be an important fuel for certain types of immune cells. Athletes who participate in prolonged, strenuous exercise have an elevated risk of contracting viral and bacterial infections. There is evidence that immune system cells are less able to mount a defense against infections after such exercise. For example, in one study at the Los Angeles Marathon, the number of athletes who became ill after the race was almost sixfold higher than non-participating athletes with a similar level of training. A number of studies have shown that a wide variety of immune responses are negatively altered by heavy training. Although there are a number of nutrients that appear to have a beneficial effect on the immune system, one of the most important appears to be glutamine.

In another study, 200 runners and rowers consumed either a glutamine-containing drink or a placebo drink. The percentage of athletes who subsequently reported no infections was 81 percent in the gluta-mine group and 49 percent in the placebo group. The author of the study suggested that supplementation with glutamine increases the availabil-ity of glutamine for key cells of the immune system.

Glutamine levels have been shown to decrease in relation to severe exercise and overtraining. Athletes who are on the verge of overtraining will probably benefit from supplementation with a protein such as whey, which contains a high percentage of glutamine.

HMB (beta-hydroxy-beta-methylbutyrate)

Beta-hydroxy-beta-methylbutyrate (HMB) is a compound that is found naturally in various foods and is produced in the body from proteins that contain the amino acid leucine. There is some evidence that HMB reduces muscle protein breakdown following exercise. Many strength and speed athletes use HMB supplements in the belief that HMB reduces recovery time and allows them to exercise more intensely, resulting in greater gains in muscle size and strength.

HMB has been widely studied. Initial research found that daily sup-plementation of HMB along with resistance training could increase mus-cle mass, reduce body fat, and increase strength in a dose-dependent manner (the more taken, the stronger the effect). More recent studies, however, suggest that HMB supplementation has no effect on strength and muscle gains. So the case for HMB is still open. Fortunately, there are no reports of negative side effects associated with HMB supplemen-tation.

Vitamin C

Vitamin C is perhaps the most multitasking nutrient in humans. It is the only vitamin that is present in every cell of the body. On a structural level, it is a major ingredient of collagen, a protein that connects cells to form tissues. Vitamin C is also a potent antioxidant that neutralizes free radicals before they can damage lipid cells. Free-radical damage is a major factor in aging and in the development of many degenerative dis-eases such as cancer.

Vitamin C helps replenish supplies of vitamin E, another important antioxidant. It also assists iron absorption and fat metabolism. Also, new evidence suggests that vitamin C supplementation may blunt the release of the catabolic hormone cortisol during especially hard workouts. Ultramarathon runners who took 1,000 milligrams of supplemental vitamin C per day for the seven days preceding a 90-kilometer run exhibited 30 percent lower cortisol levels immediately after the race and therefore very likely experienced much less muscle tissue breakdown.

Vitamin C also protects the body against viral and bacterial infections, of which athletes in heavy training are at greater risk. Daily supplementation of 600 milligrams of vitamin C significantly reduced the incidence of upper respiratory infections in individuals who participated in a marathon. In another study, an antioxidant combination consisting of vitamin C, vitamin E, and beta-carotene was found to decrease upper respiratory infections by almost 40 percent.

Because exercise greatly increases the body's use of oxygen, which is a free radical, athletes use more vitamin C to neutralize free radicals than sedentary people and therefore require more vitamin C in their diet. It is also a good idea to use a sports drink that contains vitamin C during exercise.

A daily intake of 800–2,000 milligrams of vitamin C is recommended for active adults. Exceeding this dosage may result in a number of side effects, including diarrhea and joint pain. Good sources of vitamin C include many fruits (such as oranges, grapefruit, and strawberries) and vegetables (such as tomatoes, broccoli, green and red bell peppers, and leafy greens).

Vitamin E

Vitamin E is a fat-soluble vitamin that comes in eight forms, the most prevalent and useful of which is alpha-tocopherol. Vitamin E is a powerful antioxidant. It protects cells, including muscle cells, from destruction at the hands of free radicals by helping maintain cell membrane integrity. This protection accelerates post-workout recovery in three ways: 1) it limits the loss of muscle proteins, 2) it lessens post-workout inflammation, and 3) it reduces post-workout muscle soreness.

In one recent study, thirty-two healthy men were randomly assigned to take a daily 1,000 IU vitamin E supplement or a placebo for twelve weeks and ran downhill (which causes more muscle damage than flat running) for forty-five minutes at 75 percent VO_2max, once before and once following supplementation. Blood samples were obtained before and immediately after exercise, and at six, twenty-four, and seventy-two hours postexercise. The researchers found that vitamin E supplementation had a statistically significant beneficial effect on exercise-induced muscle damage.

Several studies have also shown that vitamin E supplementation has a beneficial effect on the immune system. Whether it does so directly or by counteracting the immunosuppressive effects of cortisol is not known.

Interestingly, vitamin E seems to be more effective as a recovery aid when used in combination with vitamin C. These two antioxidants work synergistically. Recommended daily intake of vitamin E for athletes is 200–1,000 IU. Good sources of vitamin E include green leafy vegetables, legumes, nuts, seeds, and whole grains. Like vitamin C, vitamin E is a useful ingredient in a sports drink.

NUTRITIONAL SUPPLEMENTS THAT ARE EITHER UNSAFE, BANNED, OR BOTH

Athletes should avoid using any of the following substances. None of them is necessary for optimal performance in your sport if you train right, eat right, and practice the Performance Zone principles.

Anabolic Steroids

Anabolic androgenic steroids such as Dianabol (methandrostenolone), Winstrol (stanozolol), Deca-Durabolin (nandrolone decanoate), and the infamous THG (tetrahydrogestrinone) are simply man-made versions of the primary male sex hormone, testosterone. One of testosterone's many functions is to regulate the production of new muscle tissue, which is why taking steroids is a very effective way to increase muscle mass and strength.

However, it is unclear whether or to what degree the strength gains associated with steroid use affect performance in aerobic sports such as basketball and cycling. It is reasonable to expect that they would have a negative impact on performance in endurance sports due to the weight gain that comes with improved strength. Also, although this may sound cynical, it's likely that more endurance athletes would test positive for steroid use if steroids actually had a positive effect on performance in these sports.

Use of anabolic steroids increases production of the catabolic hormone cortisol. Consequently, when athletes stop using steroids, they lose muscle mass very quickly. While this might sound like an argument for staying on steroids, it's really an argument for not using them in the first place.

In addition to increasing cortisol production and likely being ineffective for athletes in most sports, anabolic steroids carry two major problems that make their use highly inadvisable. First, scientific research performed over the last twenty years has shown that steroid use causes a host of health problems. These problems include infertility, increased likelihood of injuries to tendons and ligaments, liver dysfunction (with oral steroids), heart disease, and stroke.

While the link between steroids and heart problems has not been definitively proven, case reports of steroid abusers have shown a frequent incidence of enlargement and weakening of the main pumping chamber of the heart, which not only makes the user aerobically very unfit, but can lead to heart disease and even heart attack. It appears that it will be only a matter of time before the link between steroids and heart problems becomes a unanimously recognized scientific fact. Furthermore, to date, no epidemiological study of the long-term effects of steroids use has been performed, so it's likely that other related health hazards are yet to be discovered.

The second major problem with anabolic steroids is that they are illegal and banned by the IOC, the NCAA, and scholastic athletic associations. To use them is to break the law, to cheat, and to bring dishonor upon oneself and one's sport.

Androstenedione

Androstenedione, or "andro" as most users call it, became an immensely popular supplement after Mark McGuire admitted to using it during his record-breaking seventy home-run season in 1998. (Andro was not banned by major league baseball at the time.) Androstenedione is a natural precursor to testosterone and was therefore believed to have a similar anabolic effect. It was also believed that, like steroids, it reduced the catabolic effects of training and thereby accelerated recovery.

It is now definitively known that andro does neither of these things. In the first randomized, double-blind, placebo-controlled study of its effects, andro was found to have no effect on strength or muscle mass during eight weeks of resistance training. What andro does quite effectively, however, is lower the level of HDL ("good" cholesterol) in the bloodstream, thus increasing the risk for arteriosclerosis.

In short, androstenedione is worse than useless. It has no benefits and carries major health risks. It is also banned by the IOC, the NCAA, and scholastic athletic associations.

Erythropoietin

Erythropoietin, or EPO, is a natural hormone produced mainly by the kidneys. It stimulates the production of red blood cells and increases the blood's ability to carry oxygen to the muscles. The greater the oxygen-carrying capacity of an athlete's blood, the greater his or her perform-ance capacity will be in events lasting longer than several minutes.

EPO is used medically to maintain healthy blood in patients whose red blood cell production has been compromised by liver disease or chemotherapy. Endurance athletes in search of an unfair performance advantage also inject it. While effective to some degree, the use of EPO is not only banned at all levels of sport, but it is also extremely danger-ous. It thickens the blood, creating an increased risk of clotting that becomes even greater with dehydration during exercise. A number of athletes have died as a direct consequence of EPO use. Fortunately, EPO is difficult to find and purchase, but regardless, all athletes should be strongly discouraged from even trying to obtain it.

Ephedrine

Derived from the ephedra plant, ephedrine is a central nervous system stimulant that belongs to the same molecular family as amphetamines. It has long been popular as an ingredient in weight-loss pills because it increases the rate of metabolism. It also works as a nasal decongestant. Many athletes who are concerned about their weight, including wres-tlers, gymnasts, and some football players, use ephedrine for weight loss, while others use it as an ergogenic aid (that is, to stimulate energy production).

However, there is no good evidence that ephedrine can boost ath-letic performance in any sport, and it is also dangerous. In recent years, a number of athletes have died and hundreds have become seriously ill as a result of ephedrine use. Dangerously high blood pressure, irregular heartbeat, and other serious side effects can occur in ephedrine-sensitive people, in those who overdose, and in those who combine ephedrine use and overexertion, especially in hot weather.

The Food and Drug Administration recently banned ephedrine

because of its serious health risks. It is also banned by the IOC, the NCAA, and scholastic athletic associations, and with good reason. It is a risky supplement.

Glycerol

Glycerol is a natural compound that is similar in chemical structure to alcohol. It is present in the body in stored fat and in fluids. One effect of ingesting glycerol is an increase in blood plasma volume, which is potentially beneficial to athletes because it could slow dehydration during exercise.

Studies of the effects of pre-exercise glycerol supplementation on athletic performance have produced mixed results. There is now general agreement that glycerol can increase endurance, but only in athletes who fail to drink enough before and during exercise. Since athletes should always hydrate adequately before and during exercise, glycerol supplementation is not necessary. Side effects including headaches and blurred vision are associated with excessive glycerol intake.

L-Carnitine

A natural compound with both vitamin-like and amino acid–like properties, L-carnitine is supplied in the diet by meats and is also manufactured in the liver and kidneys. Its primary function in the body is to transport fatty acids across cell membranes so that they can be metabolized in the mitochondria. L-carnitine is used medicinally in the treatment of conditions such as Alzheimer's disease and is also a popular weight-loss supplement. Some endurance athletes also use it in the belief that it can increase the body's fat-burning efficiency during exercise and thus spare the body's carbohydrate stores.

However, studies have repeatedly shown that L-carnitine supplementation has no effect on fat utilization either at rest or during exercise and no effect on endurance performance. While L-carnitine is essential for fat utilization during exercise, it appears that athletes get as much as they need in the diet and that supplementation offers no additional benefit.

Ribose

Ribose is a sugar that the body produces through glucose metabolism and is in turn used to replenish ATP stores in muscle cells. Therefore, it plays an important role in muscle energy production. Many body-builders and strength athletes use ribose supplements in the belief that they accelerate muscle recovery by increasing the rate of ATP synthesis after workouts.

However, studies have demonstrated unequivocally that ribose does not have this effect. For example, in a double-blind, randomized, placebo-controlled Belgian study, subjects performed an intensive regimen of lower-body strength exercises over a six-day period. Subjects who took a ribose supplement neither replenished ATP stores faster than placebo subjects nor outperformed them in the strength tests.

SUMMARY

Countless products that claim to enhance athletic performance are available over the counter and by prescription. Since use of many of these products is banned by various sports governing bodies and they often have dangerous side effects, it is vitally important that athletes of all ages learn the true effects and legal status of any sports supplement they are considering taking. Incorporating the principles of the Performance Zone into your training will allow you to achieve significant improvement in athletic performance simply by consuming the proper amounts of carbohydrates, protein, and water. Some of the other products that may offer benefits in terms of performance and recovery include vitamin E, vitamin C, branched chain amino acids, glutamine, and creatine.

Conclusion

n the introduction to this book we described a quiet revolution that is taking place in leading sports science laboratories around the world. It is a revolution that will change our approach to sports nutrition. Researchers are finding powerful evidence that consuming the right types of nutrients before, during, and after exercise can significantly improve athletic performance.

Sports nutrition is about to embark on a new era based on studies showing that by adding the right timing to the right combination of nutrients, athletes can perform at a higher level with greater endurance and faster recovery so they can have a stronger workout the next time. Each month new studies appear that reinforce the importance of nutrition within the Performance Zone.

Although this research has been widely published, most serious athletes and their coaches still have not incorporated the findings into their training programs. Our objective in writing *The Performance Zone* was to remove the information disconnect between the exercise science laboratories and the fields, gyms, rinks, courts, roads, and pools where athletes perform. We recognize that few areas of sport are surrounded with as much controversy and myths as nutrition. We have tried to puncture the myths and also to make it easy for athletes at all levels to use the latest sports nutrition science in their daily training by distilling it into a few basic principles that all athletes can use.

The Performance Zone was also written to counter the cynicism that many athletes and non-athletes today have regarding the best way to improve athletic performance. Each day the news media bring us frequent revelations about the use of illegal steroids and other performance-enhancing drugs by top athletes in all sports. This is unfortunate because the many studies that form the basis of this book show that drugs are not needed. We hope this book has made it clear that the most powerful performance-enhancing tool available to athletes is the food they eat.

Glossary

Adaptation. A physiological or biochemical change that occurs when the body is exposed to repeated bouts of exercise.

Adenosine triphosphate (ATP). *See* ATP.

Adrenaline. *See* Epinephrine.

Aerobic metabolism. The process of energy production that occurs in the mitochondria and requires the presence of oxygen.

Amino acids. The biochemical building blocks of proteins. There are twenty amino acids, eleven of which are nonessential and can be manufactured by the body, and nine of which are essential and cannot be manufactured by the body, so they must be supplied through diet.

Anabolism. The process of building up of body tissue and fuel stores.

Anaerobic metabolism. The process by which energy is produced that does not require the presence of oxygen.

Anaerobic threshold. The exercise intensity beyond which lactic acid begins to rapidly accumulate in the working muscles, hastening exhaustion.

ATP. Adenosine triphosphate; a high-energy compound that is the fundamental source of energy for muscle contractions.

Branched-chain amino acids (BCAAs). Essential amino acids that inhibit muscle protein breakdown and aid in muscle glycogen storage. The BCAAs are valine, leucine, and isoleucine.

Calorie. A unit of energy-producing potential that is contained in food and released during aerobic metabolism.

Capillaries. Tiny blood vessels that allow for the exchange of gases and nutrients between blood and tissue cells.

Carbohydrate. A broad category of organic compounds that are contained in food and serve as a major energy source in the body, especially during exercise.

Catabolism. The process of breaking down the body tissues, particularly skeletal muscle.

Cellular respiration. *See* Aerobic metabolism.

Cortisol. A catabolic hormone that breaks down muscle proteins for use as an energy source. It is released during strenuous exercise or when blood glucose drops below normal levels.

Creatine phosphate (CP). A high-energy compound that is stored in muscle cells in small amounts and provides a quick energy source for high-intensity anaerobic exercise or work.

Dehydration. A state in which the amount of water in the body has diminished below the level needed for optimal athletic performance.

Electrolytes. Mineral nutrients (sodium, chloride, magnesium, and potassium) that aid muscle contraction, nerve impulse transmission, and other biochemical processes.

Endurance. The ability to sustain work or resist fatigue.

Enzyme. A protein that promotes one or more types of chemical reaction in the body without itself being altered.

Epinephrine. A hormone that stimulates liver and muscle glycogen breakdown. Also called adrenaline.

Ergogenic aid. Anything that enhances physical performance. Sports drinks and energy bars and gels are considered ergogenic aids.

Fatigue. The inability to continue to work or exercise.

Fatty acid. The components of fat that are used by the body for energy.

Free radicals. Highly reactive chemicals that damage body tissues by pilfering electrons in order to improve their own stability.

Fructose. Known as "fruit sugar" because it is the type of sugar that is most abundant in fruit. It is sweeter and not as easily digested as glucose.

Glucose. A simple sugar derived from the breakdown of dietary carbohydrate that serves as a major energy fuel.

Glutamine. The most abundant amino acid in the body; especially abundant in skeletal muscles. Glutamine can be converted to glucose and used for energy and is also important for immune function.

Glycemic index. A measure of how different foods affect blood glucose levels relative to ingestion of pure glucose.

Glycogen. The form in which glucose is stored in the muscles and liver.

Glycolysis. One of two forms of anaerobic energy production, in which glycogen is metabolized without oxygen. Also referred to as the "glycolytic pathway."

Insulin. A hormone that is secreted by the pancreas; it stimulates the transport of glucose and amino acids into muscle and promotes glycogen storage and protein synthesis.

Insulin resistance. When the muscles' response to insulin is less than normal.

Insulin sensitivity. Describes the manner in which the muscles respond to insulin. A decrease in insulin sensitivity is the same as an increase in insulin resistance, whereas an increase in insulin sensitivity means the muscle response is greater than normal.

Lactate threshold. An intensity level of exercise above which the metabolic waste product lactic acid accumulates in the blood faster than the circulatory system can remove it. Also known as the "anaerobic threshold."

Lactic acid (lactate). A byproduct of anaerobic metabolism and a fuel for aerobic metabolism.

Macronutrients. The three essential nutrient types (excluding water) that are present in great abundance in the body: carbohydrate, fat, and protein.

Maltodextrin. A complex carbohydrate that is used in many ergogenic aids (sports drinks, carbohydrate gels, and energy bars) because it is easily digested.

Mitochondria. Structures within cells that serve as the sites of aerobic metabolism.

Muscle fiber. A long, thin, single cell within a muscle that is capable of contracting to produce force.

Muscular endurance. The ability of the muscles to avoid fatigue.

Norepinephrine. A hormone that stimulates heart rate and metabolic reactions. Also called noradrenaline.

Placebo. An inactive substance usually provided in a manner identical to an active substance to test for real versus imagined effects.

Protein. The fundamental structural components of all living cells and many bioactive substances such as enzymes, hormones, and antibodies. Proteins are composed of amino acids.

Recovery. A process wherein one or more systems of the body return to a normal state following exertion.

Ribose. A simple sugar found in cells. It is involved in the production of nucleotides, which are needed to produce ATP.

Simple carbohydrate. A carbohydrate with a relatively basic molecular structure.

Sucrose. Ordinary table sugar. A common ingredient in sports drinks because it is quickly metabolized to provide fast energy.

Sugar. Another name for a simple carbohydrate.

Testosterone. A hormone that is responsible for many secondary male sexual characteristics and also facilitates muscle growth.

Vitamin. Any of a number of fat-soluble or water-soluble organic substances obtained from plant and animal foods that are essential for normal biological functioning.

VO_2max. The maximum rate at which a given athlete can consume oxygen. The higher an athlete's VO2 max, the faster he or she can run, swim, bike, and so on without accumulating excess lactic acid in the working muscles.

Whey protein. A source of amino acids derived from milk.

Selected References

Anthony, J.C., Anthony, T.G., and Layman, D.K., "Leucine supplementation enhances skeletal muscle recovery in rats following exercise," *Journal of Nutrition*, 129: 1102–1106, 1999.

Armstrong, R., "Biochemistry: Energy liberation and use," IN: *Sports Medicine and Physiology*. Ed. Strauss, R. Philadelphia: W.B. Saunders, 1979.

Bell, D.G., and McLellan, T.M., "Exercise endurance 1, 3, and 6 h after caffeine ingestion in caffeine users and nonusers," *Journal of Applied Physiology*, 93: 1227–1234, 2002.

Biolo, G., Tipton, K.D., Klein, S., et al., "An abundant supply of amino acids enhances the metabolic effect of exercise on muscle protein," *American Journal of Physiology*, 273: E122–E119, 1997.

Bishop, N.C., Blannin, A.K., Rand, L., et al., "Effects of carbohydrate and fluid intake on the blood leukocyte responses to prolonged cycling," *International Journal of Sport Medicine*, 17: 26–27, 1999.

Bishop, N.C., Blannin, A.K., Rand, L., et al., "The effects of carbohydrate supplementation on neutrophil degranulation responses to prolonged cycling," *International Journal of Sport Medicine*, 21(Suppl 1): S73, 2000.

Bishop, N.C., Blannin, A.K., Walsh, N.P., et al., "Nutritional aspects of immunosuppression in athletes," *Sport Medicine*, 28: 151–176, 1999.

Blom, P.C.S., Høstmark, A.T., Vaage, O., et al., "Effect of different post-exercise sugar diets on the rate of muscle glycogen synthesis," *Medicine and Science in Sports and Exercise*, 19: 491–496, 1987.

Blomstrand, E., and Saltin B., "BCAA intake affects protein metabolism in muscle after but not during exercise in human," *American Journal of Physiology*, 28: E365–E374, 2001.

Blomstrand, E., Hassmen, P., Ekblom, B., and Newsholme, E.A., "Administration of branched chain amino acids during sustained exercise: effects on performance and on plasma concentration of some amino acids," *European Journal of Applied Physiology and Occupational Physiology*, 63: 83–88, 1991.

Bloom, W., and Fawcett, D.W., *A Textbook of Histology*. Philadelphia: W.B. Saunders, Co. 1975.

Bowtell, J.L., Gelly, K., Jackman, M.L., et al., "Effect of oral glutamine on whole body carbohydrate storage during recovery from exhaustive exercise," *Journal of Applied Physiology*, 86: 1770–1777, 1999.

Brooks, G.A., Fahey, T.D., White, T.P., and Baldwin, K.M., *Exercise Physiology: Human Bioenergetics and Its Applications* (3rd edition), Mountain View, CA: Mayfield Publishing Co., 2000.

Bruce, C.R., Anderson, M.E., Fraser, S.F., et al., "Enhancement of 2000-m rowing performance after caffeine ingestion," *Medicine and Science in Sports and Exercise*, 32: 1958–1963, 2000.

Burke, L.M., Kiens, B. and Ivy, J.L. "Carbohydrate and fat for training and recovery," *Journal of Sport Sciences*, 22: 15-20, 2004.

Cardillo, C., Kilcoyne, C.M., Nambi, S.S., et al., "Vasodilator response to systemic but not to local hyperinsulemia in the human forearm," *Hypertension*, 34: E12–E13, 1999.

Castell, L.M., and Newsholme, E.A., "The effects of oral glutamine supplementation on athletes after prolonged, exhaustive exercise," *Nutrition*, 13: 738–742, 1997.

Clark, M.W., Wallis, M.D., Barrett, E.J., et al., "Blood flow and muscle metabolism: a focus on insulin action," *American Journal of Physiology*, 284: E241–E258, 2003.

Coombes, J.S., and McNaughton, L.R., "Effects of branched-chain amino acid supplementation on serum creatine kinase and lactate dehydrogenase after prolonged exercise," *Journal of Sports Medicine and Physical Fitness*, 40: 240–246, 2000.

Costill, D.L., Dalsky, G.P., and Fink, W.J., "Effects of caffeine ingestion on metabolism and exercise performance," *Medicine and Science in Sports*, 10: 155–158, 1978.

Coyle, E.F. "Fluid and fuel intake during exercise," *Journal of Sports Sciences*, 22: 39-55, 2004.

Coyle, E.F., Coggan, A.R., Hemmert, M.K., and Ivy, J.L. "Muscle glycogen utilization during prolonged strenuous exercsie when fed carbohydrate," *Journal of Applied Physiology*, 61: 165–172, 1986.

Coyle, E.F., Feltner, M.E., Kautz, S.A., et al., "Physiological and biomechanical factors associated with elite endurance cycling performance," *Medicine and Science in Sports Exercise*, 23: 93–107, 1991.

Dangin, M., Boirie, Y., Garcia-Rodenas, C., Gachon, P., Fauquant, J., Callier, P., Ballevre, O., Beaufrere, B., "The digestion rate of protein is an independent regulating factor of postprandial protein retention," *American Journal of Physiology*, 280: E340–E348, 2001.

Davis, J.M., Zhao, Z., Stock, H.S., et al., "Central nervous system effects of caffeine and adenosine on fatigue" *American Journal of Physiology*, 284: R399–R404, 2003.

Esmarck, B., Andersen, J.L., Olsen, S., et al., "Timing of postexercise protein intake is important for muscle hypertrophy with resistance training in elderly humans," *Journal of Physiology*, 535: 301–311, 2001.

Gleeson, M., Blannin, A.K., Walsh, N.P., et al., "Effect of low and high carbohydrate diets on the plasma glutamine and circulating leukocyte responses to exercise," *International Journal of Sport Medicine*, 8: 49–59, 1998.

Gleeson, M., Lancaster, G.I., and Bishop, N.C., "Nutritional strategies to minimize exercise-induced immunosuppression in athletes," *Canadian Journal of Applied Physiology*, 26 (Suppl): S23–S35, 2001.

Gollnick, P., "Metabolism of substances: energy substrate metabolism during exercise and as modified by training," *Federation Proceedings*, 44: 353–356, 1985.

Gollnick, P.D., and Hermansen, L., "Biochemical adaptations to exercise: anaerobic metabolism," IN: *Exercise and Sport Sciences Reviews*, Vol. 1. J.H. Wilmore (Ed.). New York: Academic Press, 1973, p. 143.

Hargreaves, M., Costill, D.L., Coggan, A.R., et al., "Effect of carbohydrate feedings on muscle glycogen utilization and exercise performance," *Medicine and Science in Sport and Exercise*, 16: 219–225, 1984.

Hermansen, L., Hultman, E., and Saltin, B., "Muscle glycogen during prolonged severe exercise," *Acta Physiologica Scandanavic*, 71: 129–139, 1967.

Holloszy, J.O., "Biochemical adaptations to exercise: aerobic metabolism," IN: *Exercise and Sport Sciences Reviews*, Vol. 1. J H. Wilmore (Ed.). New York: Academic Press, 1973, p. 4471.

Hurst, T.L., Bailey, D.M., Powell, J.R., et al., "Immune function changes in downhill running subjects following ascorbic acid supplementation," *Medicine and Science in Sports and Exercise*, 33(Suppl 5): S35, 2001.

Ivy, J.L., "Dietary strategies to promote glycogen synthesis after exercise," *Canadian Journal of Applied Physiology*, 26 (Suppl): S236–245, 2001.

Ivy, J.L., "Exercise physiology and adaptations to training," IN: *Handbook of Exercise in Diabetes*. N. Ruberman (Ed.) American Diabetes Association, 2002, pp. 23–62.

Ivy, J.L., "Optimization of glycogen stores," IN: *Encyclopaedia of Sports Medicine: Nutrition in Sports*. (Ed.) S. Knuttgen. Blackwell Science Ltd. Oxford, UK, 2000, pp. 97–111.

Ivy, J.L., Costill, D.L., Fink, W.J., and Lower, R.W., "Influence of caffeine and carbohydrate feedings on endurance performance," *Medicine and Science in Sports*, 11: 6–11, 1979.

Ivy, J.L., Goforth, H.W., Jr., Damon, B.M., et al., "Early post exercise muscle glycogen recovery is enhanced with a carbohydrate/protein supplement," *Journal of Applied Physiology*, 93: 1337–1344, 2002.

Ivy, J.L., Katz, A.L., Cutler, C.L., et al., "Muscle glycogen synthesis after exercise: effect of time on carbohydrate ingestion," *Journal of Applied Physiology*, 64: 1480–1485, 1988.

Ivy, J.L., Lee, M.C., Brozinick, J.T., et al., "Muscle glycogen storage after different amounts of carbohydrate ingestion," *Journal of Applied Physiology*, 65: 2018–2023, 1988.

Ivy, J.L., Res, P.T., Sprague, R.C., et al., "Effect of carbohydrate-protein supplement on endurance performance during exercise of varying intensity," *International Journal of Sport Nutrition and Exercise Metabolism*, 13: 388–401, 2003.

Ivy, J. and Portman, R., *Nutrient Timing*, North Bergen, NJ: Basic Health Publications, 2004.

Ivy, J.L., Withers, R.T., VanHandel, P.J., Elger, D.E., and Costill, D.L., "Muscle respiratory capacity and fiber type as determinants of the lactate threshold," *Journal of Applied Physiology*, 48: 523–527, 1980.

Jun, T., and Wennmalm, A., "NO-dependent and –independent elevation of plasma levels of insulin and glucose in rats by L-arginine," *British Journal of Pharmacology*, 113: 345–348, 1994.

Kalliokoski, K.K., Kemppainen, J., Larmola, K., et al., "Muscle blood flow and flow heterogeneity during exercise studied with positron emission tomography in humans," *European Journal of Applied Physiology*, 83: 395–401, 2000.

Karlsson, J., "Lactate and phosphagen concentrations in working muscle of man," *Acta Physiologica Scandinavaca*, 358 (Suppl): 1–72, 1971.

Kingsbury, K.J., Kay, L., and Hjelm, M., "Contrasting plasma free amino acid patterns in elite athletes: association with fatigue and infection," British Journal of Sports Medicine, 32: 25–32, 1998.

Laakso, M., Edelman, S.V., Brechtel, G., et al., "Decreased effect of insulin to stimulate skeletal muscle blood flow in obese men: a novel mechanism for insulin release," Journal of Clinical Investigation. 85: 1844–1852, 1990.

Leatt, P.B. and Jacobs, I. "Effect of glucose polymer ingestion on glycogen depletion during a soccer match," Canadian Journal of Sports Science, 14:122–126, 1989.

Levenhagen, D.K., Carr, C., Carlson, M.G., et al., "Postexercise protein intake enhances whole-body and leg protein accretion in humans," Medicine and Science in Sports and Exercise, 34: 828–837, 2002.

Levenhagen, D.K., Gresham, J.D., Carlson, M.G., et al., "Post exercise nutrient intake timing in humans is critical to recovery of leg glucose and protein homeostasis," American Journal Physiology, 280: E982–E993, 2001.

Levenhagen, D.K., Gresham, J.D., Carlson, M.G., et al., "Postexercise nutrient intake timing in humans is critical to recovery of leg glucose and protein homeostasis," American Journal of Physiology, 280: E982–E993, 2001.

MacLean, D.A., Graham, T.E., and Saltin, B., "Branched-chain amino acids augment ammonia metabolism while attenuating protein breakdown during exercise," American Journal of Physiology, 267: E1010–1022, 1994.

McArdle, W.D., Katch, F.I., and Katch, V.L., Exercise Physiology, Energy, Nutrition, and Human Performance (3rd edition), Philadelphia: Lea & Febiger, 1991.

Miller, S.L., Tipton, K.D., Chinkes, D.L., et al., "Independent and combined effects of amino acids and glucose after resistance exercise," Medicine and Science in Sports and Exercise, 35: 449–455, 2003.

Miller, W.J., Sherman, W.M., and Ivy, J.L., "Effect of strength training on glucose tolerance and post glucose insulin response," Medicine and Science in Sports and Exercise, 16: 539–543, 1984.

Muckle, D.S. "Glucose syrup ingestion and team performance in soccer," British Journal of Sports Medicine, 7:340–346, 1973.

Nehlsen-Cannarella, S.L., Fagoaga, O.R., Neiman, D.C., et al., "Carbohydrate and the cytokine response to 2.5 hours of running," Journal of Applied Physiology, 82: 1662–1667, 1997.

Nieman, D.C., "Nutrition, exercise, and immune system function," IN: Clinicals in Sports Medicine, Nutritional Aspects of Exercise. Eds. Wheeler, K.B. and Lombardo, J.A., 18: 537–538, 1999.

Nieman, D.C., Johansen, L.M., Lee, J.W., et al., "Infectious episodes in runners before and after the Los Angeles Marathon," Journal of Sports Medicine and Physical Fitness, 30: 316–328, 1990.

Nissen, S., Sharp, R., Ray, M., et al., "Effect of leucine metabolite beta-hydroxy-beta-methylbutyrate on muscle metabolism during resistance-exercise training," Journal of Applied Physiology, 81: 2095–2104, 1996.

O'Connor, P.M.J., Kimball S.R., Suryawan, A., et al., "Regulation of translation initiation by insulin and amino acids in skeletal muscle of neonatal pigs," *American Journal of Physiology*, 285: E40–E53, 2003.

Okamura, K., Doi, T., Hamada, K., et al., "Effect of amino acid and glucose administration during postexercise recovery on protein kinetics in dogs," *American Journal of Physiology*, 272: E1023–E1030, 1997.

Peters, E.M., Anderson, R., and Theron, A.J., "Attenuation of increase in circulating cortisol and enhancement of the acute phase protein response in vitamin C-supplemented ultra-marathoners," *International Journal of Sports Medicine*, 22: 120–126, 2001.

Peters, E.M., Goetzsche, J.M., Grobbelaar, B., et al., "Vitamin C supplementation reduces the incidence of post-race symptoms of upper respiratory tract in ultramarathon runner," *American Journal of Clinical Nutrition*, 57: 170–174, 1993.

Phillips, S.M., Tipton, K.D., Aarsland, S.E., et al., "Mixed muscle protein synthesis and breakdown after resistance exercise in humans," *American Journal of Physiology*, 273: E99–E107, 1997.

Ready, S.L., Seifert, J., Burke, E., "Effect of two sports drinks on muscle tissue stress and performance," *Medicine and Science in Sports and Exercise*, 31(5): S119, 1999.

Rennie, M., Ahmed, A., Khogali, S.E., et al., "Glutamine metabolism and transport in skeletal muscle and heart and their clinical relevance," *Journal of Nutrition*, 126: 1142S–1149S, 1996.

Rokitzki, L., Logeman, E., Sagredos, A.N., et al., "Lipid peroxidation and antioxidant vitamins under extreme endurance stress," *Acta Physiologica Scandinavacia*, 151: 149–158, 1994.

Rokitzki, L., Logemann, E., Huber, G., et al., "Alpha-tocopherol supplementation in racing cyclists during extreme endurance training," *International Journal of Sport Nutrition*, 4: 253–264, 1994.

Sacheck, J.M., and Blumberg, J.B., "Role of vitamin E and oxidative stress in exercise," *Nutrition*, 17: 809–14, 2001.

Saltin, B., Henriksson, J., Nyaard, E., et al., "Fiber types and metabolic potentials of skeletal muscles in sedentary man and endurance runners." IN: *The Marathon: Physiological, Medical, Epidemiological, and Psychological Studies, Annals of the New York Academy of Sciences*, Vol. 301. P. Milvy (Ed.). New York, NY, 1977, pp. 3–29.

Saunders, M.J., and Kane, M.D. "The effect of a 4:1 ratio carbohydrate/protein beverage on prolonged exercise performance and subsequent recovery," presented at the Southeast Regional Conference of the American College of Sports Medicine, 2003.

Shirreffs, S.M., Armstrong, L.E. and Cheuvront, S.N., "Fluid and electrolyte needs for preparation and recovery from training and competition," *Journal of Sports Sciences*, 22: 57–63, 2004.

Spiller, G.A., Jensen, C.D., Pattison, T.S., et al., "Effect of protein dose on serum glucose and insulin response to sugars," *American Journal of Clinical Nutrition*, 46: 474–481, 1987.

Suzuki, M., Doi, T., Lee, S.J., et al., "Effect of meal timing after resistance exercise on hind limb muscle mass and fat accumulation in trained rats," *Journal of Nutritional Science and Vitaminology*, 45: 401–409, 1999.

Tarnopolsky, M.A., "Protein and physical performance," *Current Opinions on Clinical Nutrition and Metabolic Care*, 2: 533–537, 1999.

Tarnopolsky, M.A., Atkinson, S.A., MacDougall, J.D., et al., "Whole body leucine metabolism during and after resistance exercise in fed humans," *Medicine and Science in Sports and Exercise*, 23: 326–333, 1991.

Tarnopolsky, M.A., Bosman, M., MacDonald, J.R., et al., "Post exercise protein-carbohydrate and carbohydrate supplements increase muscle glycogen in men and women," *Journal of Applied Physiology*, 83: 1877–1883, 1997.

Tarnopolsky, M.A., MacDougall, J.D., Atkinson, S.A., "Influence of protein intake and training status on nitrogen balance and lean body mass," *Journal of Applied Physiology*, 64: 187–193, 1988.

Thompson, D., Williams, C., McGregor, S.J., et al., "Prolonged vitamin C supplementation and recovery from demanding exercise," *International Journal of Sport Nutrition and Exercise Metabolism*, 11: 466–481, 2001.

van der Schoor, P., van Hall, G., Saris, W.H.M., et al., "Ingestion of protein hydrolysate prevents the post-exercise reduction in plasma glutamate," *International Journal of Sports Medicine*, 18: S115, 1997.

Van Loon, L.J., Kruijshoop, M., Verhagen, H., et al., "Ingestion of protein hydrolysate and amino acid-carbohydrate mixtures increases post exercise plasma insulin responses in men," *Journal of Nutrition*, 130: 2508–2513, 2000.

Van Loon, L.J., Saris, W.H.M., Kruijshoop, M., et al., "Maximizing post exercise muscle glycogen synthesis: carbohydrate supplementation and the application of amino acid or protein hydrolysate mixtures," *American Journal of Clinical Nutrition*, 72: 106–111, 2000.

Van Loon, L.J.C., Saris, W.H.M., Verhagen, H., et al., "Plasma insulin responses following the ingestion of different amino acid and/or protein mixtures with carbohydrate," *American Journal of Clinical Nutrition*, 72: 96–105, 2000.

Varnier, M., Leese, G.P., Thompson, J., et al., "Stimulatory effect of glutamine on glycogen accumulation in human skeletal muscle," *American Journal of Physiology*, 269: E309–E315, 1995.

Williams, M., Ivy, J., Raven, P., "Effects of recovery drinks after prolonged glycogen-depletion exercise," *Medicine and Science in Sports and Exercise*, 31(5):S124, 1999.

Williams, M.B., Raven, P.B., Donovan L.F., et al., "Effects of recovery beverage on glycogen restoration and endurance exercise performance," *Journal of Strength and Conditioning Research*, 17: 12–19, 2003.

Wilmore, J. H., and Costill, D.L., *Training for Sport and Activity. The Physiological Basis of the Conditioning Process* (3rd edition), Dubuque, IA: Wm. C. Brown Publishers, 1988.

Wolfe, R.R., "Effects of amino acid intake on anabolic processes," *Canadian Journal of Applied Physiology*, 26: S220–S227, 2001.

Yaspelkis, B.B., Patterson, J.G., Anderla, P.A., et al., "Carbohydrate supplementation spares muscle glycogen during variable-intensity exercise," *Journal of Applied Physiology*, 75: 1477–1485, 1993.

Zawadzki, K.M., Yaspelkis, B.B., III, and Ivy, J.L., "Carbohydrate-protein complex increases the rate of muscle glycogen storage after exercise," *Journal of Applied Physiology*, 72: 1854–1859, 1992.

Index

About the Authors

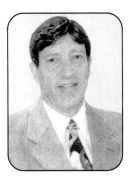

John Ivy is Chair and Margie Gurley Seay Centennial Professor in the Department of Kinesiology & Health Education at the University of Texas at Austin. He received his Ph.D. in Exercise Physiology from the University of Maryland and his post-doctoral training in physiology and biochemistry from Washington University School of Medicine. He has published over 150 research papers on the effects of nutrition on physical performance and exercise recovery. He is a Fellow and former Ambassador for the American College of Sports Medicine and Fellow in the American Academy of Kinesiology.

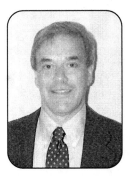

Robert Portman earned his Ph.D. in biochemistry from Virginia Tech. He has numerous scientific publications and has written and lectured extensively on the role of nutrition in improving exercise performance. Dr. Portman is head of research at PacificHealth Laboratories, a nutrition technology company that has pioneered in the development of innovative nutritional products to help athletes reach their potential.

Drs. Ivy and Portman are coauthors of *Nutrient Timing: The Future of Sports Nutrition* (Basic Health Publications, 2004).

ALSO FROM BASIC HEALTH PUBLICATIONS

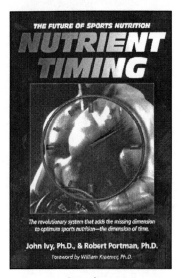

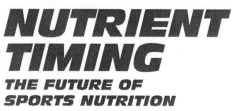

THE FUTURE OF SPORTS NUTRITION

John Ivy, Ph.D., & Robert Portman, Ph.D.

Foreword by William Kraemer, Ph.D.

If you are serious about weight training, you have probably experienced the "plateau phenomenon." You train harder, you consume extra protein in your diet, but you just don't get the strength and power gains that you want. For the last ten years sports nutrition has focused on *what* to eat. The latest research from leading sports science labs now shows that *when* you eat may be even more important. *Nutrient Timing* adds the missing dimension to sports nutrition, the dimension of time. By timing specific nutrition to your muscle's 24-hour growth cycle, you can activate your body's natural anabolic agents to increase muscle growth and gain greater muscle mass than you ever thought possible. *Nutrient Timing* is the biggest advance in sports nutrition in over a decade.

By applying the principles of the Nutrient Timing System, you'll be able to deliver the precise amounts of nutrients needed at precisely the right time to optimize your muscle-building agents and maximize muscle growth, while minimizing muscle damage and soreness after a hard workout. You'll even be less susceptible to colds. You can actually sculpt a better body with more lean muscle mass, less fat, and more power without changing your exercise program or even your total caloric intake. *Nutrient Timing* will show you how.

"*Nutrient Timing* represents the next important nutrition concept in the 21st Century."
—**WILLIAM KRAEMER**, PH.D., PROFESSOR, UNIVERSITY OF CONNECTICUT

"Drs. Ivy and Portman take sports nutrition to a new level. A must read for the strength coach and athlete."
—**MICHAEL STONE**, PH.D., HEAD, SPORTS PHYSIOLOGY, U.S. OLYMPIC COMMITTEE

US $14.95/Can. $23.95 • 6 x 9 Quality Paperback • Health/Nutrition/Fitness • ISBN 1-59120-141-1

Available at bookstores and health food stores everywhere.
Visit www.basichealthpub.com or call toll free 1-800-575-8890 to order.

Y 613.2 IVY
Ivy, John,
The performance zone :
R2001932660 MILTON

ODC

Atlanta-Fulton Public Library

CPSIA information can be obtained at www.ICGtesting.com
Printed in the USA
BVOW081738201212

308770BV00004B/8/P

9 781591 201489